Praise for *Letting t[...]*

"Philip M. Berk's personal story de   ⌐⌐⌐cer and the suffering it entailed is beautiful and compelling. His story will open you to an increased understanding of the awesome healing power of guided imagery, visualization, dream work, meditation, and emotional expression. He wonderfully illustrates how a strong spiritual connection is the source of all healing. *Letting the Light In* offers clear, useful, authentic, and heartfelt practical advice for the benefit of all."

—Dr. Candace Pert, Ph.D.,
author of *Everything You Need to Know to Feel Go(o)d*

"While living in challenging and uncertain times, Philip M. Berk inspires us on how to keep our light shining... Philip's work is brilliant."

—Sandra Ingerman,
author of *Medicine for the Earth*

"*Letting the Light In* is an inspiring account of crisis, healing, and transformation. It is a classic hero's journey in which Philip Berk faces death, acquires great wisdom, survives, and returns to share with others what he has learned. This is a wonderful account of the transformative power of love and letting go."

—Larry Dossey, MD, author of *Healing Words*
and *Prayer Is Good Medicine*

"What an inspiring and magical book! Philip M. Berk's poignant story can teach every one of us to be genuinely grateful for even the most serious challenges that we face."

—Jeff Levin, Ph.D.,
author of *God, Faith, and Health*

"A much needed perspective on how to embrace suffering as part of life's experience. A must read."

—Judith Cornell, Ph.D. [Rajita Sivananda],
award-winning author of *Mandala: Luminous
Symbols for Healing* and recipient of six
Lloyd Symington awards to empower those
challenged by cancer to receive the spiritual
and emotional support they need

Letting the Light In

About the Author

Philip M. Berk (Oregon) is a certified Reiki Master and healer, a cancer survivor, an educator, a writer, and a holistic therapist.

To Write to the Author

If you wish to contact the author or would like more information about this book, please write to the author in care of Llewellyn Worldwide and we will forward your request. Both the author and publisher appreciate hearing from you and learning of your enjoyment of this book and how it has helped you. Llewellyn Worldwide cannot guarantee that every letter written to the author can be answered, but all will be forwarded. Please write to:

Philip M. Berk
ᶜ/ₒ Llewellyn Worldwide
2143 Wooddale Drive
Woodbury, MN 55125-2989, U.S.A.

Please enclose a self-addressed stamped envelope for reply,
or $1.00 to cover costs. If outside the U.S.A., enclose
an international postal reply coupon.

Many of Llewellyn's authors have websites with additional information and resources. For more information, please visit our website at:

www.llewellyn.com

Letting the Light In

Transforming Your Pain Into Power

Philip M. Berk

Llewellyn Publications
Woodbury, Minnesota

First Edition
First Printing, 2010

Cover design by Lisa Novak
Cover image © Digital Stock Tranquility
Text quoted on pages 100, 101, and 135 is taken from *Left to Tell:
    Discovering God Amidst the Rwandan Holocaust* by Immaculée
    Ilibagiza © 2006 with permission of the publisher Hay House Inc.,
    Carlsbad, CA.

Llewellyn is a registered trademark of Llewellyn Worldwide, Ltd.

Library of Congress Cataloging-in-Publication Data
Berk, Philip M., 1974–
Letting the light in: transforming your pain into power / Philip M.
Berk.—1st ed.
    p. cm.
  Includes bibliographical references.
  ISBN 978-0-7387-1973-3
  1. Spiritual life. 2. Suffering—Religious aspects. 3. Berk, Philip M.,
1974– 4. Testis—Cancer—Religious aspects. I. Title.
  BL65.S85B47 2010
  204'.42—dc22

                                                    2009054086

Llewellyn Worldwide does not participate in, endorse, or have any authority or
responsibility concerning private business transactions between our authors and
the public.
  All mail addressed to the author is forwarded but the publisher cannot, unless
specifically instructed by the author, give out an address or phone number.
  Any Internet references contained in this work are current at publication time,
but the publisher cannot guarantee that a specific location will continue to be
maintained. Please refer to the publisher's website for links to authors' websites
and other sources.

Llewellyn Publications
A Division of Llewellyn Worldwide, Ltd.
2143 Wooddale Drive
Woodbury, MN 55125-2989, U.S.A.
www.llewellyn.com

Printed in the United States of America

This book is dedicated to Alexis Treulieb,
my wife and spiritual companion,
whose radiant love enlightens my soul.

CONTENTS

ACKNOWLEDGMENTS

Letting the Light In has been an incredible journey filled with so many blessings and so much love. This journey was only possible because of the amazing support of so many wonderful people in my life. First and foremost is my wife, who helped guide so much of this work. She not only spent her time helping me edit my manuscript and further my ideas, but continually nourished me with her unconditional love. Her sweet love is the only reason that I have been able to reach inside to find the strength and confidence to transform myself. She is such an incredible human being. She is the sweetest, most humble, intelligent, wise, and compassionate person I have ever known. I am so honored to share my journey of life with her. My daughter has also been an unbelievable source of strength for me. Her beautiful spirit has blessed my life with so much light and I feel so grateful to be her daddy. Her miraculous presence has renewed my heart and helped me to believe in the power of love to heal my life. She is such a beautiful and radiant little girl! My mother's support has also been absolutely amazing and deeply touching. There is no one else in the world that I can rely on like her. Time after time she flew out to be with my family and me during my surgeries and chemotherapy sessions. She is my rock. She is my foundation. She has always believed in me and I am forever indebted to her. From the time I was a little boy, she has always nourished my spirit with a belief that I could achieve anything that I desired. She continues to teach and guide me. She is the most giving, caring, and thoughtful person I have ever known. Her unwavering support and unconditional love has helped me in ways that I cannot put into words. My sister has also been a huge support in my life. She has always been there for me. Together we share an enormous bond of friendship that is a major healing force in my life. She has always offered me wise and deeply caring advice and has always nurtured my spirit with tenderness and love. Her sense of humor, comforting warmth, and profound inner strength are an inspiration to me. She helps me in countless ways and I feel blessed to have her by my side. I am also indebted to my father who recently passed away. My father was an esteemed guru of the literary world who inspired me to write from an early age. My father's passion for the arts has blessed my life immeasurably. He taught me how important it is to fill my life with my own personal bliss, passion, and meaning. He taught me that nothing is more important than living an authentic and genuine life. He continues to guide me. I feel his love all the time and I know that this work is infused with so much of his wisdom that he passed on to me.

I thank my agent Anita Kushen for her continual belief in myself and my work and her steady and persistent commitment to making this book a success. I also thank my acquisitions editor, Carrie Obry, for believing in this work and helping me to make my dream a reality. I thank Ed Day, my production editor, who helped fine-tune my manuscript.

There are so many more family and friends I wish to thank. I would like to thank Dennisha, Bob, Eva, Marlene, Harriett, Elizabeth, Sarah, Jonah, Isaac, Adam, Beverly, Frank, Grandma Iva, Joyce, Taya, Kelly, Dr. Audrey Siow, Dr. Andy Swanson, Dr. Tony Murczek and the Soaring Crane Qigong Group, Ida Bauer and the entire CU Family Development Center, Sante from Penrose Hospital, Jessica, Jay, Mina, Dennis, Crystaline, Phyllis, Lecia, JeeYun, Bodhi, Jason, Courtney, Koko, Grandpa Arty, Aunt Linda, Uncle Steve, Uncle Danny, and the entire New Seasons Concordia crew.

INTRODUCTION

It was almost six years ago that I sat in my hospital bed watching Lance Armstrong win his record-breaking Tour de France. Since at the time I was also going through testicular cancer, I felt a special interest in watching Lance power his way through to another amazing victory. During his "victory ride," while he rode down the Champs Élysées in Paris, I started thinking about when my own victory ride would be. At that precise moment, while watching the hospital TV set, I started to get a very uncomfortable feeling inside my chest, wondering if there would even be a victory ride. Here I stood, attached to an IV with extremely intense chemotherapy drugs flowing through my veins twenty-four hours a day, my hair, my eyebrows, my eyelashes completely gone, my energy fully depleted, and my life force vanishing right before my eyes. I started to feel an enormous fear that penetrated the very core of my being—a fear that spoke of loss and death and desperation and loneliness. At twenty-nine years old, I felt like I was spiraling downward into death instead of thriving and living my life. I felt caught, stuck, confused, and lost.

This fear was not new to me. In fact, this fear has almost always guided every aspect of my life. The fear took many forms—insecurity, anxiety, embarrassment, isolation. It seemed as though my heart was continually paralyzed, my mind permanently disabled, my will to live completely exhausted. As I was lying down that morning thinking about my freedom of life without cancer—my own personal "victory ride"—I began to imagine a new life, a new me, a life lived without continual fear and anxiety. What would this new life look like? What would this new me be like?

At the time of my cancer diagnosis, I had spent almost half my life burdened by an emotional and physical trauma that obviously helped create the testicular cancer that I was now facing. When I was fourteen years old, I was diagnosed with undescended testicles and needed surgery to correct them. After the surgery, I was given weekly testosterone shots. I was also told that I would be infertile for the rest of my life. These experiences wounded my sense of self. They made me feel like I would always be inadequate and never fully be a man. Every day from then on was filled with shame and embarrassment, insecurity and humiliation. I lived life without any self-confidence, self-love, or self-worth. Every relationship was experienced through a need to feel approved, every decision was made with a need to be recognized, every moment was infused with a desperate

and unhealthy need to know that despite my inner discomfort I was somehow okay—but I was far from okay,
and I knew it.

I felt isolated from all that was good. I felt that goodness wasn't for me—that somehow I didn't deserve it. I
felt that because of my traumatic experiences I would
always be tainted and imperfect, and thus unable to receive the abundance that comes from living a life filled
with an inner presence of health and wholeness. All of
my energy thus far had been spent resisting instead of
embracing life, struggling with instead of accepting myself, and doubting the power of Spirit instead of trusting in it.

While I was sick with cancer, I was able to confront
the harsh and unhealthy way I had been living my life.
When someone tells you that you could die, you begin
to fight for your life. So I started examining the inner
thoughts, feelings, and images that had defined my inner world—and what I began to see in every darkened
place I looked was one thing—fear.

I was scared of life, myself, my experiences—but most
of all I was scared of love. How could this be? How could I
be scared of the one thing that I needed most? As I started
to recognize this disequilibrium in my life, I became extremely curious about why I was so scared of something
that was so good for me. This curiosity started me on a
journey of reading that began with modern New Age
books on health and healing and led me all the way into
ancient spiritual texts. Everything I had read, from the

stories of the Buddha to Jesus, from Moses to Saint Francis, illustrated the same message, only worded differently. This message was *Let yourself and your fear go and let in the healing and divine power of love.* I began to understand that once I was able to let go of my continual fear and receive this great love, I would heal my life. This love is the source of all miracles, it is the power that heals the body, mind, and spirit, and it is the pure and untainted energy of Spirit. When you awaken this love, you awaken the presence of Spirit—and when Spirit awakens within, you become completely transformed.

I wanted nothing more than to welcome this holy transformation into my life—but how? How could I break free of the prison of doubt and fear that had become my life? Upon facing this seemingly insurmountable situation with an urgency to change, I quickly realized that in order to change my life, it only made sense that I would have to change myself. So I began examining myself, not with disdain and embarrassment as I had done for the better part of my life, but with curiosity and mindfulness—and by doing so, I actually began to befriend myself. This shift was enormous. I became very comfortable with my own company, something I hadn't felt since I was a child. An even bigger achievement was that I became comfortable enough to examine my own fear. I started doing artwork, especially writing. I enrolled in yoga classes. I began to meditate. Very quickly I learned how to face my fear and myself with openness and ease, rather than the harsh resistance that I had become so used to.

This refocusing of my energy from resistance to openness, from fear to love, is the reason that I am now a healthy person. Once I made the decision to face my biggest fears, my fears eventually dissipated. And I believe that once my fears dissipated, my cancer also left my body and my life for good. There is more joy in my life now than I could have ever imagined. The experience of illness was the catalyst for this awakening and I am very grateful for these experiences.

Directly after my experiences with cancer, I made the decision that I would always focus my energy on health and healing. I began to take my writing practice more seriously by dedicating a portion of time every day to write about spirituality and the healing process. A lot of my early writing was poetry, the form I was most comfortable with. Many of these poems are included throughout *Letting the Light In*. This poetry was my first motion toward making sense and meaning of the challenging experiences I had endured. It was also one of the first ways I had learned to communicate with my soul and connect with and express spiritual truth.

As well as developing a serious writing practice, I also became a certified Reiki Master and a professional mental health therapist. During this time period, I developed my own system of healing. My system of healing is based on my own experience with life's many challenges.

What I know for a fact is that all of life's challenges can be successfully harnessed so that the magic of healing can unfold. This magic happens through breaking down resistance and allowing an opening for the healing light to come in. This is why I have termed the seven steps of my healing system as gateways. Gateways are simply openings—a way in where there once wasn't.

My work as a healer and therapist focuses on exploring how to break open the built-up resistance within ourselves. I use many wonderful exercises to relax the body and mind, work with the breath, release emotions, connect with the power of intention, perform healing ceremonies, and develop the healing presence of inner joy and peace. I have found that once you are able to open all the blocked passageways in yourself, you are led into a brilliant and divine landscape filled with overflowing possibility, personal power, and spiritual transformation.

Exactly two years after my last chemotherapy session, during which I was pondering my own "victory ride," I had the opportunity to travel to Paris to honor the passing of my father. By chance, on the very first day of our trip we ventured down the Champs Élysées and spotted the Arc de Triomphe. Looking up at the beautiful structure, I instantly remembered my moments in the hospital watching Lance Armstrong win his historic seventh victory. With an emphatic "Yes!" I ran up the many stairs to the very top, and once I was at the top, I looked over the gorgeous city with a feeling of complete renewal. I had done it! I had completely transformed myself. I felt so much gratitude for life. I felt so much love for myself. I felt completely overwhelmed by the power and beauty of Spirit. I knew at that moment that with Spirit, with love, anything was possible.

There is a light in this world, a
healing spirit more powerful than
any darkness we may encounter.
We sometimes lose sight of this force
when there is too much suffering,
too much pain. Then suddenly, the
spirit will emerge through the lives of
ordinary people who hear a call and
answer in extraordinary ways.

—MOTHER TERESA

ACCEPTANCE

IN THIS VERY MOMENT
*you hold the key to overcoming
every obstacle, unfolding every
blessing, and discovering the infinite
possibility of love and life.*

It was sunrise and I can still remember the way the sky's vibrant colors filled my shocked and bewildered eyes. The streaks of orange and gold against the backdrop of the majestic Rocky Mountains were the first touch of grace that began my new life.

I had just spent the entire night in the emergency room doing endless rounds of ultrasounds, blood tests, and x-rays. I knew something was not right when I went to the hospital that night—but I had no idea it was cancer. It made no sense to me. Most people say that when they are stunned by life in this way, it feels like you are inside a dream—or, for that matter, in somebody else's life. That's exactly how it felt.

On my way home from the hospital, I could hardly drive. Every two to three minutes I would start shaking and crying uncontrollably. I remember screaming at the top of my lungs, "No! ... Please! ... I want to live ... Please!" I had to pull over to the side of the road because I was crying so hard that I was gasping for air—almost choking. I happened to stop right next to a park. I sat in my car trying to calm myself down. I was in no condition to go home and tell my wife the news.

Music was something that had always calmed me down. I turned on the radio in my car and continued watching the sunrise while listening, slowly calming myself down. The second or third song that came on the radio was "The Velvet Glove" by the Red Hot Chili Peppers. The song seemed to be talking directly to me. I will never forget when Anthony Kiedis sang about disasters being a star falling in his yard.

It pierced me to the core.

It took me many years to fully understand and internalize what this meant. I struggled for many days and nights with the idea that what was happening to me, the "disaster" of cancer, was actually a blessing—a "star falling in my yard." For quite some time, I felt that this unbearable hardship was nothing but a nuisance and a horrible barrier in my life. That was my mindset even though there were so many people I talked to that emphatically told me that their unique personal challenges were "the best thing that ever happened to me." They told me that "if I gave myself away to the challenge before me, I would transcend all my personal limitations and barriers." I didn't quite understand.

In my desperation and loneliness, I often retreated into a depression that would last many long days and nights. The depression was marked by an overwhelming feeling of despair. This despair was filled with continual thoughts of helplessness. I felt helpless in the face of this enormous challenge. I felt helpless in the face of my continual anxiety and fear. I felt helpless in the face of my years of trauma and emotional dysfunction. I felt helpless because that was all I ever knew how to feel.

As my journey with cancer unfolded I was pushed forward, over and over again, into an overwhelming feeling of urgency. I was continually forced to face this despair and helplessness, even though I really just wanted to be left alone. But I knew that in order to heal my life—in order to stay alive—I was going to need to change. No matter what tactics I tried to pull to hide from myself and my life, nothing seemed to work. I had avoided dealing with myself at all costs. I smoked marijuana every chance I could get. I changed jobs as quickly as I got them. I even used spiritual practices such as *kirtan* (ecstatic chanting) to escape rather than deal with my life. But when cancer appeared, I knew I could no longer sustain these dysfunctional patterns. In every place I turned to try and escape, I was always brought back to the one urgent and critical question: "What are you going to do to change your life?"

Even though I struggled most of the way, I eventually learned to embrace and accept my experience with testicular cancer. The challenge of cancer forced me to face myself. It forced me to look deep within my soul for answers. It begged and pleaded for me to face my biggest fears. And it screamed and howled for me to let go of my continual self-loathing and to finally learn to love myself.

I finally understood what everyone meant when they said that their experience of life's challenges were "the best thing that ever happened." I learned that they are the "best thing" because they force you to wake up to the blessing of your life. Without my experiences with life's immense challenges, I would still be living my life half asleep. Without these experiences, I would still be spending my time stuck in fear instead of living with love.

Marianne Williamson, internationally acclaimed author and lecturer, states: "The darkness is an invitation to light, calling forth the spirit in all of us.... Can you reach within yourself for enough clarity, strength, forgiveness, serenity, love, patience, and faith to turn this around? That's the spiritual meaning of every situation: not what happens to us, but what we do with what happens to us and who we decide to become because of what happens to us."

It is only through life's challenges that you are presented with the opportunity to transform and heal yourself. This is because your challenges create an opening in your life to work with your suffering. What stops most people from transforming themselves is the unwillingness to accept and engage this powerful energy. Your suffering is the fuel for spiritual awakening, because your suffering is what opens your heart and reveals you to your soul. It is only through a complete breaking open of your heart that the essence and meaning of your life is unfolded. This journey inward has been called "the hero's (or heroine's) journey." This journey into darkness, into your pain and discomfort, is one you must make if you are to awaken the light of your soul and heal every part of your life.

Acceptance of Suffering

Throughout time, the experience of embracing and accepting one's suffering has been the path to profound spiritual awakenings. Prince Siddhartha, also known as Gautama Buddha, was first led on his journey of awakening through the experience of suffering. Since he was a prince and lived in a palace, he was never confronted with the harshness of life. It wasn't until he had left his palace as a young man that he saw that life was not just luxury and comfort, but also hardship and difficulty.

On his journey into the nearby village, he encountered people whose lives were filled with intense suffering. He saw a crippled man, a decaying corpse, and many people who were stricken with disease. Upon seeing this suffering, he realized that by being so sheltered in his palace, he had not come in contact with the true nature of life.

As he came in contact with this suffering, he decided to abandon his entire inheritance, give up all his possessions, and live an authentic life committed to spiritual practice. He was compelled to learn how to transform his suffering and the suffering of others into the healing ground for awakening. What the Buddha eventually realized was that all of life—including our suffering and bliss, our pain and pleasure—needed to be accepted and compassionately worked with.

In Herman Hesse's book *Siddhartha*, a fictional portrayal of the story of the Buddha, he describes this realization in further detail: "It seems to me that everything that exists is good—death as well as life, sin as well as holiness, wisdom as well as folly. Everything is necessary, everything needs only my agreement, my assent, my loving understanding; then all is well with me and nothing can harm me."

Saint Francis of Assisi is another example of a great saint who transformed his suffering into the means for a spiritual awakening. Francesco, as he was first called, was the son of wealthy parents and, like Prince Siddhartha, had lived a life of comfort. It wasn't until he went off to war as a young man that he came in contact with suffering. He saw many of his friends die and was also taken as a prisoner of war.

When he returned to Assisi a year later, he was stricken with a serious illness that began his spiritual awakening. Coping with this illness allowed him to see into the fallacy of his previous existence and eventually propelled him forward into an authentic life.

He, too, decided to give up all his riches, his jovial nights drinking with his friends, and his family's honor to lead a life dedicated to truth and authenticity. During the time of his illness, he realized what was important and what was not. He saw that worldly possessions were nothing compared to the wealth of the Spirit. From that point on he vowed to live a life that honored this tremendous realization.

The examples of Saint Francis and Gautama Buddha are just two examples of the many people throughout history that have allowed the experience of suffering to transform their lives. Only through the experience of suffering can you become a wiser and stronger human being. Thich Nhat Hanh's eloquent words further illustrate the way in which suffering can help you grow:

> Without suffering, you cannot grow. Without suffering, you cannot get the peace and joy you deserve. Please don't run away from your suffering. Embrace it and cherish it. With understanding and compassion, you will be able to heal the wounds in your heart, and the wounds in the world. The Buddha called suffering a Holy Truth, because our suffering has the capacity of showing us the path to liberation. Embrace your suffering, and let it reveal to you the way to peace.

I never had experienced suffering the way I did during my prolonged stays in the hospital. Not only was I experiencing intense suffering in myself, but I also saw it everywhere around me. The hospital setting was a continual reminder that I was not the only one suffering—the whole world was suffering. I saw everything from innocent children suffering with leukemia to elderly people recovering from strokes and heart attacks and cancer to young people who had been rushed to the emergency room after automobile accidents.

My own suffering made me even more aware of other people's suffering. Observing the suffering of others helped me to willingly step out of my comfort zones and accept the experience of suffering as a part of my life experience. For many years I was devoted to an idea about myself that, despite my early trauma when I was fourteen years old, I was perfectly fine and healthy. I had spent my entire twenties running away from myself. Escaping from my life is what I did best. I believe I moved every year for over seven straight years. I couldn't sit still, because I knew that if I sat still long enough I would be confronted with the reality of my suffering—and at the time I wanted nothing to do with it. My comfort zones were to escape. During this time I maintained a very juvenile attitude that suggested that whenever things got challenging or difficult in my life I should "just bail." I had a "whatever—I don't care" motto that suggested that my life and life in general were not to be taken seriously. The culmination of this time period is when I lived on the beach in Hawaii. For over six months, I didn't work, I didn't live in a house, I hardly contacted any friends or family, and I did absolutely nothing but try to forget my life. I was dirty, hungry, and alone. I remember one day, after taking a shower at a nearby campground, I took a glance at myself in the mirror and was astonished by what I saw. Not only did I see a lost and confused young hippie, but I saw a sadness, a suffering inside myself that made me step back and away from the mirror.

When I was diagnosed with cancer at age twenty-eight I knew I couldn't run anymore. I was forced to sit still and deal with and try to accept my wounded self. I was forced into seeing, feeling, and experiencing an intense and unbearable suffering within myself. My experiences with chemotherapy continued to bring me into the darkest of places, continued to challenge me to face and accept the rawness of this suffering.

There was one night in particular when I felt swallowed in the darkness. I felt like Jonah in the belly of the whale, confronted with the severity of my pain and inner turmoil. This night was the Friday after one of the many weeklong hospital stays. Fridays were always the worst as I would feel the week's accumulation of chemotherapy drugs rushing through my body, which made me feel so horrible. This night, unlike most other nights, I couldn't stop throwing up. I felt dehydrated and delirious, dizzy and lightheaded. But I didn't want to wake up my wife in the middle of the night. I also didn't want to go back to the hospital, because I had developed a serious loathing to being there. So I thought I would stick it out. I spent most of the evening curled up in a ball in the middle of the living room. Internally I knew what was happening—I was battling all my demons, all my fears. Externally, I was scared for my life. Even though it is hard to remember exactly what happened that night, I remember repeatedly saying, "Here I am … Here I am … Here I am." I remember telling death and suffering that I was not afraid and that I fully accepted them. I remember by the end of the night I had changed positions from a tight, clenched-up ball to lying prostrate on the floor with my arms spread wide open. At this point in the night, I was calling out my wife's name and eventually, when I saw her standing above me, I felt like I had returned from the darkness of the belly of the whale and was back on shore, safe again. By the looks of me, though, I don't believe that she thought I was safe, as she immediately called an ambulance. I spent the next three days in the hospital.

One of the most important things I have learned is that by staying present and open, even when you are in the midst of tremendous pain and are scared to the brim of your suffering, you develop a tremendous fearlessness that affirms the great power that lives deep inside. If you remain scared and hide in what you know and what is comfortable instead of facing your suffering, you fail to grow and learn and develop this courageous life-affirming attitude. The biggest and foremost barrier that blocks the ability to accept and courageously face your life is the very easy tendency to stay in your comfort zones.

Comfort zones rob you of life's power. They like to trick you into thinking that you can make your life easy and pain free. They distract you from facing your difficulties and your pain. They imprison your spirit and take away your freedom to live life with conviction and power. The experience that I previously mentioned easily could have been just a very hard night of being sick, but because I allowed myself to fully embrace my suffering, I learned something very important about myself. I learned that I could deal with whatever came my way—death, suffering, sorrow, pain. Most importantly, I learned that I could live my life without fear.

Comfort zones are the places that we remain when we would rather not deal with our suffering and instead protect ourselves from dealing with this aspect of our lives. There are many ways we hide and escape from facing the rawness of our life experience. We may numb ourselves with too much TV, intoxicants, or work. We may numb ourselves by never sitting still long enough to face ourselves. We can become so emotionally disinterested that we forget how to fully connect with ourselves, each other, and the presence of Spirit. This resistance is the root of our spiritual dysfunction. This resistance is what forces us to be afraid of life instead of embracing it.

When you are not able to open yourself to what life offers you, you create an insurmountable barrier between yourself and your experience. This barrier expresses itself in many ways, but the thread running through each way will always be stress. Stress is the direct outcome of not letting go. Stress is brought about when you cannot accept yourself, your life, and the moment at hand. Stress is your body and mind's response to the unwillingness to face your life.

The only way to let go of your fear, resistance, and subsequent stress is to willingly step forward and face it. This takes a tremendous amount of courage to allow yourself to be open and vulnerable to what hurts and challenges you. Once you make the decision to embrace your suffering, though, you instantly bless yourself with great courage and inner strength and will be turned into a warrior. A warrior lives life fearlessly. No matter what happens, no matter how threatening the unknown looks and feels, a warrior uses every last bit of personal life experience to facilitate self-improvement. Everything becomes an opportunity to transform one's life. A warrior harnesses difficulty and this is what allows him or her to develop an unwavering presence that is not based on fear.

In the eloquent words of the late psychiatrist and author Elisabeth Kubler Ross: "You will not grow if you sit in a beautiful flower garden, but you will grow if you are sick, if you are in pain, if you experience losses, and if you do not put your head in the sand, but take the pain as a gift to you with a very, very specific purpose." This purpose is to transform yourself into someone who lives life completely open to each and every life experience, knowing that every experience can be harnessed, every moment can be uplifted, and every day can be a living testimony to the great power that lives within.

Acceptance of the Life Process

Life is always testing us, always pushing us, always challenging us to grow—to move beyond our limitations. This is the nature of life and the life process. Everything that is alive must engage in ongoing change and transformation. Otherwise, we are simply not living. In "It's Alright Ma (I'm Only Bleeding)," Bob Dylan noted that people who resist change are already dying. I believe that this observation reveals the extreme openness we must have in order to fully accept and engage in every aspect of the life process.

Whatever the challenge may be, whatever the difficulty, we must allow it to open us to change—to push us out of whatever has become too rigid and stagnant in our lives. In the words of one of my favorite poets, Rainer Maria Rilke: "What locks itself in sameness has congealed. Is it safer to be gray and numb? What turns hard becomes rigid and is easily shattered. Pour yourself out like a fountain."

This process is the movement from from dis-ease to ease, from disequilibrium to equilibrium, from disharmony to harmony. We are always moving in and out of this process. We are always in a constant state of becoming. We never arrive at a place where we do not have to face the challenge of self-transformation. Self-transformation is our continual task.

Life is a process made up of endless patterns and relationships of change that continually evolve and grow.

With an Awareness

Of death
Each breath
Transforms itself
Into a gateway
To fully experience
Each new day
Where each moment
Becomes a little
More precious
Like a lover's last kiss
Reminding you of
The fleeting nature
Of existence
Opening your heart
To the mystery
Of experience
Allowing you to possess
What is most important
Which is not the body
And not the things
Of this world
But the beauty
Of the Spirit
And the truth
Of the eternal

Nothing in life is ever stagnant. If something were to stop growing, it would eventually wither away and die. Life's challenges are the part of the process that propels you forward into change and thus help to keep you fully alive and fully engaged with every part of your life. Without emotional, mental, physical, and spiritual challenges, you would never grow. The experience of these challenges propels you into this new growth and thus it may be the most important and fulfilling aspect of the life process.

The life process can be likened to that of the seasons. In spring there is new life, in summer there is a culmination of that life, in autumn that life undergoes a major transformation, and in winter that life regenerates itself and passes. In order to be a healthy individual, you must incorporate the full spectrum of this process. There is beauty in the death of winter just as there is in the spring of new life. There is beauty in the ease and playfulness of summer just as there is in the transformation and letting go of autumn.

Once you are able to see life as an experience of endless change rather than something you try to control and own, you will be able to let go of all your resistance and truly live your life. The reason change is so frightening is because of the state of groundlessness you experience when you decide to fully engage in the life process. By giving yourself to the raw and wild experience of being alive, you realize that there is absolutely nothing to hold onto—not even yourself. Because you are always changing, you begin to see that you are not the same person you were ten years ago that you are today and that you will not be the same person in twenty years, as well. This feeling makes you question who and what you really are. You also begin to come to terms with the fact that one day you are going to die and pass into the most mysterious change of all. Living with all of this awareness is frightening, but necessary. This crucial awareness is what allows you to live your life in a genuine and honest manner.

Instead of viewing death and change in a way that disables you, you can see it as a miraculous experience— one that keeps you open and appreciative of the miracle of being alive. While it is true that life is a series of losses, it is also true that you can transform these losses into a series of gains when you choose to let go into the process of life.

The experience of change definitely sets you up to experience many losses. When I was first diagnosed with cancer, the most important thing I had lost was my "normalcy." I felt like my "normal" life was gone. I felt like the "normal" things I had taken comfort in were all stripped away. Instead of hanging out with my friends, I had appointments with doctors. Instead of thinking about what I was going to do on the weekend, I had to think about what I was going to do to release emotional trauma. Instead of sitting down to eat whatever I wanted to, I had to think about every little thing I could or couldn't eat.

For the first few weeks of all of this, I felt horribly depressed. I just wanted everything to go back to the way it was, but I knew there was no way that this was going to happen. My life had completely changed—and I knew that I needed to change with it.

One night while journaling and listening to music, I had an emotional breakthrough where, for the first time, I saw the many losses in my life as an exciting opportunity and new growth. I was listening to "Anthem" by one of my favorite musicians, Leonard Cohen, who kept singing about cracks being in everything, but also noted the positive—cracks allow light to get in. During this evening, I began to see my whole situation in a completely new way. I began to realize that the many "cracks" or losses in my life that cancer had brought with it were opportunities for the light of new things to come into being. This inner realization helped to shift my continued resistance and ongoing depression. The following weeks marked a dramatic change in the way I approached my illness. I became very excited to learn about my health and healing. I started reading books on healing the mind, body, and spirit, I began researching healthier ways to eat, I enrolled in Reiki classes, and I started to meditate.

These experiences helped me witness firsthand that by consciously shifting the focus from that of resistance to that of acceptance, you can begin to engage with life in a deeply spiritual and open way. This shift happens when you choose to let yourself go into the ever-changing rhythm of life. By letting yourself go, allowing yourself to experience the many changes that life is always presenting, you discover that it is actually the reality of impermanence that makes your life so precious.

At the first gateway, where you uncover a natural openness and acceptance in your life, you learn to accept the impermanence of life as something of great significance and value. You begin to see how incredibly precious life is and how blessed you are to be participating—it's the gift of being alive! You begin to see that the present moment is all you ever really have and that's what makes it your greatest blessing. Again, in the words of the late psychiatrist and author Elisabeth Kubler Ross: "It's only when we truly know and understand that we have a limited time on earth—and that we have no way of knowing when our time is up—that we will begin to live each day to the fullest, as if it was the only time we had."

We all are faced with the fleetingness of time. We are all going to live only a short while. A lifetime is not very long. We all have to make the decision: are we going to live this short amount of time with fear and resistance, not living the life we could have, not being the person we could have, or are we going to step forward and greet the unique chance of a lifetime with openness, acceptance, and love?

How to Enter this Gateway: Relax Your Body

Throughout time, the body has been called a temple. Within the temple of the body, you make the decision to either be open and accepting of life or rigid and closed down. Where you are at any given moment can be directly linked to how you are feeling in your body. If you are tense and stressed, you are not going to be very open. In Karlfried Graf Durckheim's enlightened book, *The Way of Transformation,* he further illustrates how important the body is in achieving an openness and acceptance of life: "The body in its posture, its patterns of tension and relaxation, in the rhythm of its breathing and manner of its movement, is an infallible indication of the point at which any person has arrived on the way to becoming a person. It may reveal how and where we are stuck … and to what extent we have remained open to our being and on the way."

The main reason we sometimes get "stuck" is because we become dismayed with life, which eventually leads to stress. Stress arises due to the inability to accept life as it is. If you are unable to accept life as it is, there is no possible way of relaxing in the present moment. This resistance to life produces an incredible amount of tension that makes it very difficult to allow healing energy into your life.

Stress is one of the biggest reasons that people get sick. It not only lowers our immune system, but it actually stops the ever-present flow of life inside the body.

In its rigidity and desperate need for control, it forces you to turn away from what you most need—which is openness and love. We often spend so much of our time focusing on such trivial matters as our finances, our work, when our car needs the next oil change, and on and on. This trivial thinking forces us to forget about our spiritual presence, which is boundless and free, and instead forces us to focus on a fear-based presence that is confused, lost, and stuck.

When you are stressed, your body becomes tense and your breath becomes shallow. This rigidity does not allow the body to heal or restore itself. If you are to heal yourself, you must first learn to relax the energy of your body. The most important aspect of relaxing your body is done through relaxing and opening your breath. Your breath is directly linked to your life force. Your life force is the spiritual energy that sustains you. In China this life force is called *chi* and in India this life force is called *prana*. Both chi and prana are the divine energy that sustains your life in every way imaginable. It is an unseen force that gives life to all things, and without it, nothing could survive. This life force is what helps everything in life continually move, grow, and evolve. When you breathe, you draw this life force into your body—and if you are not breathing correctly, you will lack the necessary nourishment to sustain your body. Keith Sherwood, one of the first pioneers in the field of natural healing, author of *The Art of Spiritual Healing*, states:

Being sick is not a static state of being. It is a process; it is fluid, continuing only as long as you nourish it. By removing your support, you can reverse the process. Once you stop feeding it, once you alter the conditions necessary to keep it going, the disease will starve and eventually disappear.

When you breathe properly, you bring nourishment and vitality into your system. The vital force (prana) helps the body mobilize its resources against disease. With greater force mobilized against it, the disease is forced to respond to less harmonious conditions within the body.

Breathing exercises have the power to relax and soothe you and release any built-up tension that is causing you to resist life. Breathing exercises also have the power to heal you. In the yogic tradition they practice *pranayama*, which is a form of breathing exercises that use the breath and certain "locks" in the body to circulate the healing energy of prana (life-force energy), which is found in highest concentrations in the air we breathe. Pranayama is a practice of storing and gathering this prana and then directing it to specific areas of the body that need healing. In many cases, breathing exercises alone have healed people from incurable diseases.

Many of us simply forget to breathe correctly—it is so simple and automatic that we figure that it is already taken care of. In our day-to-day lives, amidst all the busyness, we forget to connect with and open our breath. This causes many disturbances in both our bodies and minds—and without a relaxed and deep quality of breathing that unifies and relaxes both our bodies and minds, we will not be able to discover the peace and tranquility of the present moment.

By opening and nourishing your breath, you instantly relax your body, enter the sacredness of the present moment, and cultivate a healthy and strong life force. It is only through this relaxed and accepting presence that you will be able to open your arms to receive the present moment. In the words of cancer survivor, healer, inspirational author, and speaker Louise L. Hay, "The point of power is always in the present moment."

My experiences using breathing exercises to help me become more present and open have proven to be incredibly powerful. I can remember many difficult situations while I was sick when I used my breath to transform my anxiety and resistance into a deep sense of peace and calm. One of the hardest weeks of my life, my first week of chemotherapy, was to say the least an extremely challenging and upsetting period of time. I had spent almost ten days lying in a hospital bed, without even enough energy to get up and take a walk. My mind was quite disturbed by the drastic shift in my reality. Within three weeks I went from being in a warm and nurturing environment with my family, holding and cuddling my newborn baby, to the sterile, scary, and cold environment of the hospital. I was frightened and scared, lonely and confused. When the hospital chaplain came in to talk with me that week, I could barely utter a word to him about how I was coping—I simply wasn't.

My body was carrying more tension than I could bear. Due to the extreme emotional and physical pain, I had become completely disconnected from my body. Because all I could do was just lie there, I thought that there was absolutely nothing I could do to remedy my tension and uneasiness. Since all the methods of relaxing myself had been stripped away, I was at a loss regarding how to carry on. Then it occurred to me, being a yoga practitioner, that the corpse pose was something I could do. The corpse pose is a posture that is performed while lying down. In the past, I had used this pose to release physical tension throughout my body while practicing deep breathing. While I was lying on the hospital bed, I realized that not only could I practice the corpse pose, but I also had the most valuable tool available to me—my breath. I regularly started using my breath to release stored-up tension in my body. Every time I felt stressed out, I would scan my body to find out where I was holding this tension and then I would use the power of my breath to dislodge it. This healing practice, time and time again, would instantly relax and bring me back into my body. This connection sustained my awareness of the present moment and helped me to cultivate an ease in handling the many complexities of my situation.

Exercise: Working with the Breath

Stress and tension are the direct result of built-up resistance and fear. Stress and tension are the way your body communicates an imbalance in your body. The way to release this tension and balance your system is through the harnessing of the breath. The breath has the power to immediately dissipate all tension and replenish and rejuvenate your life force.

This exercise is done in three parts. The first part guides you to open and relax the breath, the second part allows you to use the breath to release your tension, and the last part uses the breath to refuel your energy and activate your life-force energy.

Lie down in a comfortable place where you will not be disturbed. Place both of your hands onto your stomach. First, notice the rhythm of your breathing. Is it relaxed or is it tense? Does it flow smoothly or does it flow abruptly? Does it fill you with a sense of ease or does it fill you with a sense of agitation?

If your breath is already deep and smooth, then continue breathing in this way, allowing your hands to rise and fall with each new breath. If you find that your breath is shallow and agitated, start calming the breath by breathing deeply into your abdomen. Use your hands to guide the breath going in and out of your abdomen. With each in-breath, allow your hands to rise and with each out-breath allow them to fall. Your hands should be gently guiding your breath, allowing you to breathe very deeply and smoothly.

As your breath becomes more serene and peaceful, start to visualize the ocean. Think of its rhythm and sound. For each inhale and exhale, I would like you to constrict your throat to make a sound that resembles the ocean. This will help you to deepen your breathing. As you lift your abdomen up to inhale, visualize a large wave lifting up inside the ocean. Match the size of this great wave with the full extension of your abdomen. As you exhale, visualize this wave falling and dispersing onto a sandy beach. As you visualize this wave traveling to the very end of the sandy beach, allow your exhale to be fully drawn out to match the long length that this wave would travel. Repeat this visualization until you feel that your body is fully relaxed and your breathing becomes effortless.

Secondly, once your breath is open, start taking notice of the stored-up tension located in different areas of your body. You can start scanning your body as if you were taking x-rays all the way from your head and shoulders down to your legs and feet.

Once you locate where the tension is stored in your body, start using the breath to release this tension. For example, if you find tension in your shoulders (a very common place), then breathe directly into that area of your body and continue breathing there until you feel that your shoulders have become more relaxed. On an inhale you allow your breath to embrace whatever area of your body is tense and needs attention, and on the exhale you use your breath to release this tension. If necessary, you can make a sound while exhaling, which helps some people further eliminate this tension.

Your breath works as a softening agent. Whatever feels hard and rigid, your breath softens. As you release tension in your body, you will release your emotional tension, as well. Since emotional angst, such as anxiety and worry, stores itself in your body, this exercise will greatly affect the way you feel—both emotionally and physically.

Lastly, on an inhale, visualize a golden light coming from just above your head and then traveling down your body and resting itself in your abdomen. Imagine this golden light as a bright and powerful sun of life-force energy. On your exhale, visualize this sun's vibrant light emanating and flowing from your abdomen into every cell of your body. Imagine every cell of your body receiving this golden healing warmth. Repeat this visualization for five to ten minutes until you feel fully restored.

The Message of this Gateway:
Where You Are Is Where It's At

When you no longer struggle with life, you accept it. When you no longer fight with life, you embrace it. When you no longer resist life, you free the healing power that is inside of you.

By simply accepting your life, just as it is, you free yourself from the confines of resistance and discover the freedom of being fully present. This awakened presence accepts the inevitable reality of suffering and knows that it is only through accepting and facing this reality that life becomes a miraculous journey. As you continue to live within this awakened presence, you naturally unfold an abundance of gratitude. This gratitude will open up life's healing power that is always available to you.

TRUST

WHEN YOU TRUST,
you allow yourself to let go.
When you let go,
you free yourself from doubt.
When you are free from doubt,
you become fearless.

Acceptance and trust are the groundwork for all healing that takes place in your life. While acceptance allows you to let go of resistance and relax into the process of life, trust allows you to perceive all the events in your life as experiences for growth and healing.

When you are confronted with the immensity of life's challenges, it becomes very easy to "freak out," and search outside of yourself for some reassurance that everything is going to be okay. I did this for quite some time—both before and after the experience of cancer. I was so tightly wound in an anxiety about losing everything precious to me that I couldn't be present with what life was trying teach me. Not being present with my life created an ongoing struggle in which I did not allow the power of life to support and guide me.

Trusting that life was guiding me in the face of cancer seemed counterintuitive. It seemed that my life was not right and the only way to make it right was to forcefully conquer and fix it. I spent all of my time from the diagnosis to years after being "cancer free" running around in circles trying to fix myself. The diagnosis of cancer made me feel like I had become forever tainted and broken, as if I would always be damaged goods. It seemed that from now on I would always have to be poked and prodded to make sure I was going to be all right. This severely wounded my ability to trust in my own body and mind to heal itself. Even when I was told I was "cancer free," I still felt the same overwhelming anxiety. So, in my fearful desperation, I tried almost every healing technique that had ever been created. I tried acupuncture, massages, vibe machines, fasts, supplements and herbs, prayer machines sending healing vibrations into my picture, and on and on and on. Although many of these healing techniques were wonderful, I was overdosing on them. I was doing too many things at once, because I lacked a trust in my own healing power. Due to my doubts that life would take care me, I wanted to cover all my bases—but what I was really doing was distracting myself from taking full responsibility for my healing process. In my frenzy to get to the next appointment and try the next thing, I had not allowed myself the quiet space of inner peace and stillness to listen to what life was trying to tell me.

It took many years to discover that life was trying to tell me to simply let go and trust that no matter what, I was going to be just fine. It took a lot of money spent on many healing modalities to discover that no matter what I did, I still felt the same overwhelming anxiety. This anxiety was rooted in a continual fear. I was scared of cancer, hospitals, doctors, chemotherapy, but mostly

I was scared of losing control. This fear expressed itself in many ways. I experienced asthma, headaches, dizziness, shakiness, and many other symptoms in my body. I also experienced panic attacks, obsessive thought patterns, and a continual onslaught of neurotic feelings that suggested that I was sick—that something was always wrong. What was truly wrong was that I lacked a healthy relationship to the way that I was approaching my life.

After many "freak out" sessions, I learned that this anxiety could not be healed by searching for anything outside of myself. I knew that this anxiety could only be healed by learning to change my responses to myself and to life. For this to happen, I needed to develop a relationship to cancer that was not based on fear. I had to learn to trust that the experience of cancer was exactly what I needed to heal my life. Life was offering me an opportunity for growth and renewal. I was being challenged to say "yes" to life, no matter how scary and uncertain the circumstances. This was an opportunity for me to harness the power inside myself to further my spiritual journey.

One of the most influential books in my life is Viktor Frankl's *Man's Search for Meaning*. Frankl was a Holocaust survivor who was also a psychotherapist. Because of his training, he was involved in counseling many of the prisoners at the death camps. What he found was that survival in the Holocaust often depended more on spiritual qualites than physical ones. He discovered that the people that had lost faith in life quickly deteriorated, while the people that were able to persevere with a sense of faith and trust in life were able to survive much longer. He states that this trust in life was made by an "inner decision" to choose their own responses to life. In his own words: "Even though conditions such as lack of sleep, insufficient food and various mental stresses may suggest that the inmates were bound to react in certain ways, in the final analysis it becomes clear that the sort of person the prisoner became was the result of an inner decision, and not the result of camp influences alone. Fundamentally, therefore, any man can, even under such circumstances, decide what shall become of him—mentally and spiritually."

At the second gateway, you learn how to respond to life in a trusting manner. This very important skill will allow you to unfold a mental and spiritual presence that is unmoved in the face of any difficulty or challenge. I have witnessed firsthand how changing your responses from doubt to trust can instantly change your life. This shift is achieved by examining the beliefs you hold about yourself and about life. In order to find your way back into trust, it is important to begin to examine these beliefs so that you can start to understand why you respond the way you do. In order to achieve this sense of trust, you can begin by reflecting on these questions: "Am I patient and gentle with myself?" "Do I perceive the events in my life with an attitude of surrender or do I resist them?" "Do I accept my life as it is or do I struggle with my life, believing it should be something other than what it is?"

Trusting in Life

Edvard Munch, a Norwegian painter and printmaker, once stated, "without fear and illness, I could have never accomplished all I have." Stephen Hawking, the famous modern-day physicist who has dealt with the debilitating and paralyzing illness ALS, was asked, "How do you feel about having ALS?" to which he responded, "The answer is, not a lot. I try to lead as normal a life as possible, and not think about my condition, or regret the things it prevents me from doing, which are not that many." Christopher Reeve, the famous actor who was paralyzed in an accident, once stated, "I refuse to allow a disability to determine how I live my life. I don't mean to be reckless, but setting a goal that seems a bit daunting actually is very helpful toward recovery."

I love these quotes because they remind me how important it is to face your life with an inner conviction of trust and fearlessness. They remind me that the greatest power we always hold is the ability to decide not to fight with our lives—instead we can decide to courageously work with our lives. This fearlessness stems from a belief that life will guide you no matter what. When you hold this belief inside yourself, you trust that every experience is perfect as it is—there are no accidents—and everything has a divine purpose, even your suffering.

Trusting is not an easy thing to do. It seems as though we are all mentally programmed from early on in our lives to distrust almost everything and everyone, including ourselves. We are taught not to trust neighbors, strangers, or anyone that looks different from us. We are also taught not to trust that we have the ability to take care of ourselves. We are mistakenly guided that we must consult the "experts" to figure out everything in our lives. We must read this book or consult this professor or go to that doctor to get an answer to our questions. We no longer trust our natural instincts. We no longer believe that we have a great power deep within. We no longer feel, to use part of Marianne Williamson's famous quote, that we are "powerful beyond measure."

Shifting this focus takes some willpower. It takes a willingness to want to work with the "monkey mind," which is always focused on trying to manipulate the external world to receive some kind of internal gratification. This false identification with life creates an enormous barrier to learning how to trust in ourselves. It tries to trick us into thinking that we must control everything that happens to us. Oftentimes, it is within the moments of crisis that our innate ability to trust is awakened. In those moments when there are no answers, when the "experts" cannot provide the solutions, when the mind cannot comprehend, and the outside world is out of control, we are left with a choice. We can either open ourselves to the unknown and trust in the life process or face it in despair.

When I was first undergoing treatments for testicular cancer, I had to learn how to let go of control and trust that life would guide and support me, even when the onslaught of bad news seemed endless. No matter what the doctors told me, I felt I was always receiving the worst news possible. After my first surgery, doctors told me that I had a 50 percent chance of a recurrence. A year later, this chance became a reality. After undergoing three rounds of chemotherapy, I was told that I had a 95 percent chance that the cancer in my lymph nodes would be gone. However, the chemotherapy had not affected the tumor at all. After the chemotherapy, I agreed to have a six-hour surgery to remove the lymph nodes from the base of my spine. I was reassured that there was an 80 percent chance that no further treatment would be necessary. The tumor was perhaps not malignant. A few days later, I learned that it was malignant. Two more rounds of chemotherapy were ordered—both of which were to be intensified significantly beyond the original dosage.

After each round of bad news, I would sink into a horrible depression where I remember repeatedly saying and thinking that if there was a higher power in life, it obviously didn't care about me. I felt forsaken. I felt that no matter what I did or didn't do, I was always left feeling hopeless and lost. I was stuck in endless worry and doubt. I decided, "Why should I trust in life when all life wants to do is make me feel horrible and sick?" During one of my stays at the hospital, the hospital chaplain visited me. No matter what the chaplain said, he couldn't get through to me. I remember how sad his eyes were as he listened to my ongoing self-pity. Then he took a Bible out of his brown leather bag and read a few different passages. The passages that I still remember him saying were, "Though he slay me, yet I will trust in him," and "If you can believe; all things are possible to him who believeth." I remember him repeatedly telling me to "trust in life even though it was challenging me" and to "be patient because there will be a redemption."

I know that for quite some time I held a belief that life was supposed to be perfect—and anything short of perfection meant something was wrong. I also believed that life was supposed to be easy and pain free. I believed if things weren't right in your life, if they were filled with too much pain and suffering, you had to work forcefully against them to make them easier and less painful. One month of cancer treatments changed all of this. I didn't know what to believe anymore. At the time, I remember my mother gave me a copy of Don Miguel Ruiz's life-changing little book entitled *The Four Agreements*, in which he states that "ninety-five percent of the beliefs we have stored in our minds are nothing but lies, and we suffer because we believe these lies...You have to find the courage to break those agreements that are fear-based and claim your personal power."

These words and the words of many spiritual texts that I had started to read helped me begin to see how the beliefs that I was holding on to were strangling me. They were not allowing the mental freedom to face my life. The rigidity of what I believed life to be did not allow me to let go, trust, and learn to be patient with my experience or myself. My beliefs had created a strong impulse to fight and struggle with everything. This is because my beliefs reflected a strong fear that life was not on my side. I felt that in order to make life work for me, I had to use force to influence it. The opposite was true, though. What I really needed to create a space of healing in my life was gentleness.

At the time, my responses to life were anything but gentle. Because I perceived everything that was happening to me as an attack against me, I continually felt the need to fight. This fighting spirit wasn't the optimistic and positive one, though. This fighting spirit was born in desperation and fear. I was so scared of what my life had become. I was scared of what I might become. I was also scared that I would die and never get the chance to make my life right. Cancer had opened up all the windows and doors to my secret inner world of continual self-loathing and embarrassment and I knew that now was the time in my life to face it—but I was so scared to do it. I was caught in so much fear about how to face my life that, out of this severe discomfort and anxiety, I could not face the reality of what my life actually was. And because I couldn't face the reality of my life, I felt helpless in the immensity of it. This helplessness paralyzed me with its incessant struggling—its onslaught of anxiety and stress. I was continually struggling with the belief that my life was not right and I was impatiently waiting for it to somehow become right. *But this was my life.* The desperation, loneliness, uncertainty. I began to

LETTING GO OF CONTROL

You allow things to flow
No longer blocking
The way with resistance
Or pointless expectation
You open yourself to being
Engage with living
Give yourself to seeing
The perfection of love
In all things—
No longer caught up
In distinctions
That limits the mystery
Of creation
You open yourself
With spontaneity
You forget yourself
With humility
You bow down
Respectfully
Greeting each
New experience
As it comes
Unifying yourself
And the moment
Into one

realize that maybe life was messy—maybe life was just this—and somehow I needed to trust that it would be all right, I would be all right—everything would simply work out.

Throughout my experiences with cancer, I have learned how important it is to simply let go and trust, even when you cannot understand what it is life is presenting. This letting go of control will help you to release all the anxiety and worry that blocks your ability to trust. This anxiety is simply a disbelief that life is on your side. As soon as you let this doubt go, everything will open up for you. Again in Marianne Williamson's words: "To trust in the force that moves the universe is faith. Faith isn't blind, it's visionary. Faith is believing that the universe is on your side, and that the universe knows what it's doing. Faith is a psychological awareness of an unfolding force for good, constantly at work in all dimensions. Our attempts to direct this force only interferes with it. Our willingness to relax into it allows it to work on our behalf."

You only have one choice; you either work with life or against it. You either struggle with doubt, experiencing endless worry and inner turmoil, or you trust the spirit of life and experience endless support and guidance. The spirit of life beckons you to come forward and greet it. Once you step forward, life will take care of the rest.

Trusting in Yourself

Once you learn to trust in life, you begin to listen to what life has to tell you. Life is always trying to communicate through you. The problem is that we often don't listen to what it is trying to tell us.

In my own experience, as well as in talking to many other people who have dealt with many of life's challenges, I have found that most often these experiences are life trying to tell us about the need for further self-love, self-acceptance, and self-worth. Our challenges remind us that there is always room for more growth, more understanding, more love.

As I have already mentioned, the barrier standing in the way of embracing this transformation is the nature of your beliefs. The beliefs you cultivate either nurture or damage yourself. The beliefs you hold contain a tremendous amount of power and energy. This is because every belief you have either supports and guides your journey into health and wholeness or singlehandedly destroys it. Norman Cousins, author of *Anatomy of an Illness*, further illustrates the power of your beliefs:

> The greatest force in the human body is the natural drive of the body to heal itself—but that force is not independent of the belief system, which can translate expectation into physiological change. Nothing is more wondrous about the fifteen billion neurons in the human brain than the ability to convert thoughts, hopes, ideas and attitudes into chemical substances. Everything begins, therefore, with belief. What we believe is the most powerful option of all.

All false beliefs have roots in the unhealthy way you view yourself and your life—from a lack of self-love and self-acceptance. The most detrimental belief you can hold is that you and your life are not good enough. This belief starts from a pursuit to be perfect, in which you abandon your inner divinity and instead impose all sorts of unfair demands upon yourself. If you spend your time focusing on these self-imposed faults, you believe that you should be better than you are, that you should be prettier or more handsome, that you should be smarter, and so on and so forth. All these "shoulds" cause you to doubt yourself and believe in a false sense of self. Again in Don Miguel Ruiz's words, "We have the need to be accepted and to be loved by others, but we cannot accept and love ourselves. The more self-love we have, the less we will experience self-abuse. Self-abuse comes from self-rejection, and self-rejection comes from having an image of what it means to be perfect and never measuring up to that ideal. Our image of perfection is the reason we reject ourselves; it is why we don't accept ourselves the way we are."

A false sense of self continually tries to inform you that you do not deserve to feel good about yourself. It tries to make you believe that you are not worthy to receive love. If you get lost in this illusion, your whole life will become filled with fear instead of with love. This fear exhausts your ability to face your life with compassion and gentleness, which are absolutely necessary for your continued growth and healing.

This false sense of self also promotes many behavioral patterns that continually strip you of your power. These patterns take the form of dysfunctional and often unconscious habits that keep you from confronting life, such as overeating, smoking, drinking, doing drugs, watching too much TV, and on and on. These behaviors are sustained by the false beliefs that continually try to rob you of your energy. These beliefs live in the subconscious mind because of a trauma or series of traumas that were never fully processed. Since these traumas do not go away, they simply store themselves away and hope that someday they will be consciously acknowledged and eventually processed.

If you decide to live your life with a lack of gentleness because of your inability to create trusting belief patterns, it will be impossible to foster the necessary awareness to successfully heal these traumas and change their corresponding habitual behaviors. If you do not trust in yourself and your ability to harness your life experiences, you are quickly led into an apathy and despair that causes you to lose sight of your own self-worth. I should know; this was exactly my experience.

My self-worth became compromised due to my extreme insecurity about myself. The trauma of the surgery I experienced at the age of fourteen precipitated this insecurity. I was always beating myself up with unloving and harsh thoughts. I was always telling myself horrible things like, "You will never really be a man," or "No one will ever really want to be with you." The habitual behaviors that went along with this damaging self-criticism were passive, but destructive—I never fully gave myself to anything. Because I believed that I was not good enough for anyone or anything, I continually quit or quickly ran away from any and all of life's responsibilities. I quit a professional teaching job in the middle of the school year, told myself my school loans didn't exist, and persisted in being in a relationship with a woman who betrayed me.

The basis for this dysfunction was that I hadn't learned how to trust and love myself. Because of my emotional and physical trauma, I viewed myself as imperfect and thus somehow tainted and unfit to be loved. The fact was I hated myself. I was embarrassed and ashamed of myself. The way that I had learned to deal with myself was to not love myself or allow myself to be loved. One of the first messages that I received during my experience of cancer was to stop perpetuating this toxic attitude and behavior.

It wasn't until I got cancer that I started to look at how abusive I was being toward myself. I remember my first "wake-up call" concerning this damaging behavior. It was the third day after my last major surgery and, due to the intensity of the procedure and the many drugs I was taking, my face and body were a bit swollen.

During the middle of the night, I had gotten up to take a very difficult walk to the bathroom. While I was in the bathroom, I looked at myself in the mirror with an overwhelming feeling of negativity and disgust. I

YOU ARE A CHILD OF LIFE
Not the shadow
Of a distorted idea
Or a mistaken reality
That lost itself
In its search for an identity
Forgetting that it didn't need
To search
'Cause within you
Is a beauty and divinity
And a Spirit
That moves perfectly
It is what you see
When you truly
Open your eyes
It is what you feel
When you let go
Of all your self-doubt
And realize
It is what you become
When you are
Completely content
With what lies inside

started telling myself how ugly I was and how I could not believe that anyone would ever be attracted to me.

As I laid back down on my bed, I took a deep breath and could not believe what I had just stated about myself. I had been through hell and back and had courageously confronted all of it, and now I was telling myself such awful things. As I looked down at the many staples the doctors had put on my stomach, I began to close my eyes, put my arms around myself, and I started to pray. I prayed that I would one day start viewing myself as a beautiful man and that I would start feeling unconditional love for myself.

I fell to sleep with the prayer resting deep inside of me—and that night I received the answer to the prayer. I had a very powerful dream that helped me to begin to break through the many barriers that had stopped me from viewing myself in a healthy way.

In the dream, I was walking in the woods with a tremendous amount of baggage and discovered a very interesting temple. As I approached this temple, I saw that the door had two words engraved on it that read: "Be Thyself." Before entering the temple, I had to empty all my pockets and leave my backpack and my many bags that I was carrying around. Once I took off my backpack and let go of my three or four bags, I felt incredibly light.

As I entered, I noticed how the inside of the temple formed a mandala. There was a beautiful golden center with a large stained-glass window directly above it. The temple formed the shape of an octagon and on each side there was a stained-glass window. On each of the eight sides there was also a little meditation room, where people were meditating and praying. There was also an abundance of plants hanging from the ceiling, with vines that covered the entire temple walls.

I was instinctively drawn to go to the center where the sun was directly shining through the middle stained-glass window. As soon as I sat down, a very old and wise spiritual master emerged from one of the meditation rooms. He sat with me and looked into my eyes without blinking once. I inherently knew that I was not supposed to turn away from his gaze.

Within a few minutes of looking into his eyes, he told me, through his incredibly wise eyes, everything I needed to do to answer my prayer. Through this silence, I became aware of all the damaging statements in my mind and how they were continually taking my power away from me. I soon realized that these habitual patterns could be transformed through self-love. I realized that in order to open my heart to this unconditional love, I had to nourish myself with complete trust and self-acceptance.

After I received the spiritual master's wisdom, he closed his eyes and meditated with me for the rest of the dream. After the meditation, I opened my eyes and looked up into the stained-glass window, where the sun was still shining through. As I stared into the brilliance of the sun, I felt an overwhelming warmth surround me, and then I woke up.

This dream taught me that when you trust in yourself, you let go of any beliefs about yourself that try and dim your inner light. When you trust in yourself, you honor and respect the great power that is you.

If you believe you are not worthy of love, you will act in ways that will not draw love into your life. The only way you can begin to heal is by cultivating a space in your life for this love for yourself to exist. This love is the essence of who and what you truly are. When you trust and believe in yourself, you begin to open yourself to receive this healing presence.

How to Enter this Gateway: Relax Your Mind

At the second gateway, you realize that the mind is a garden. If you don't tend to it, spending time cultivating what you would like to grow, you will have an overgrowth of unruly weeds. These weeds are the negative thoughts that try and drain your life force. The process of tending to your garden means that you pay attention to your thoughts and work on creating a mental space that is free from negative thoughts and thus clear, spacious, relaxed, and open.

The most effective and profound way you have of nurturing your immune system is through nurturing your thoughts. The immune system is directly affected by the quality of your thinking. It is common knowledge that positive and loving thoughts make the immune system healthy and strong, while negative and disturbed thoughts stress and drain it. In the words of acclaimed author and inspiring speaker Deepak Chopra, "Every cell in your body is eavesdropping on your thoughts."

Meditation is the best way I have found to compassionately work with the mind. Not only are you able to cultivate healthy thoughts, but you are also able to develop witness consciousness. Witness consciousness is the ability to see all your thoughts, without getting attached to them. By not attaching yourself to your thoughts, you develop a sense of self that is not wrapped up in the false beliefs about life or yourself. By simply watching your thought process, you achieve an incredible amount of freedom that allows you to stop struggling.

Once you are able to objectively and compassionately step back from your thoughts and remove any unnecessary harshness or judgment that you may be placing on yourself, you will be able to see yourself with the gentleness and love that you deserve. In Wayne W. Dyer's inspiring book *Your Sacred Self,* he further illustrates witness consciousness:

> True awareness is a state of pure witnessing, without any attempt to fix or change that which is being witnessed. It is a kind of nonjudgmental love that, by itself, is healing. Even if what you observe is "sickness" or "infirmity," the compassionate witness notes the trouble spots and observes them with unconditional love. The absence of

judgment in the act of observation contributes the appropriate energy of love that the situation needs.

When I was first diagnosed with a recurrence of testicular cancer, I was in a state of continual anxiety and stress. For over a month, I was confused about what I should do. I was so consumed with my indecisiveness that I had created an incessant inner dialogue that played over and over again in my head. Some of the ongoing questions racing through my mind were:"Should I do chemotherapy or should I not? Should I go on a retreat or should I stay home? Should I quit my job and move in with my family or should I continue to work? Should I listen to this doctor or should I listen to that doctor?" And then there were the judgments and the self-loathing, which sounded something like this: "What good are you? How could you let this happen to you? You are such a mess and now you need someone else to help you clean it all up—again!"

My mind was a chaotic mess. I was unable to focus and relax. I was so disturbed by this endless chatter that I wasn't able to sleep, I could hardly eat, and I had a very hard time communicating with my friends and family members. Time was moving on and I felt like I had to make some kind of decision about what I was going to do, but I was still clueless. I slowly started to realize that if I was going to figure out the best course of action, I was going to need to quiet my mind. During this time, I used to take many walks with my wife around our

Do not wait
Meditate
And create
A healing space
Of stillness
In your heart
Create
A perfect state
Of silence
Where you start
To radiate
Love
And emanate
Peace
And give yourself away
To seeing the divinity
That lives within
All things

neighborhood. On each of our walks, we would always pass by a little creek that passed through our neighborhood. One day it occurred to me to sit by the creek and meditate. I believe I must have sat there for almost an hour. When I got up to walk home, I was amazed at how good I felt. For the first time in at least a month, my mind was clear and I didn't feel so heavy with doubt and anxiety. It didn't take long for me to see how I was clearly creating a false idea about myself and how harsh and judgmental I was being toward myself. It also didn't take long for me to realize what decision I needed to make. I knew I needed to do everything possible to regain my health. I needed to try the chemotherapy. This immediate clarity helped me to see how I was the one responsible for making myself feel depressed, confused, and insecure, and I how I was also the one responsible for making myself feel calm, centered, and confident.

Buddhist teacher and author Pema Chodron states, "Meditation practice is how we stop fighting with ourselves, how we stop struggling with circumstances, emotions, or moods." This is exactly what meditation practice and the ability to cultivate witness consciousness has done for me. By helping me separate myself from my mind's exhausting dramas, it has helped me to transform my life. This has taken the form of a very clear and awakened sense of self that no longer mistakes who and what it is.

There are many different styles of and approaches to meditating. Almost all of them focus on the breath as a way to achieve inner stillness and calm. As mentioned in the Acceptance chapter, the breath is the vehicle for awareness. It removes stress from the body and helps the mind to become clear and calm. By following your breath, you are able to pay better attention to your thoughts. By paying attention to your thoughts, you can begin to see how the quality of your thinking affects your life. As so many spiritual teachers throughout the ages have already stated—if you transform the way you think, you gradually transform your life.

I use a very simple technique during meditation that involves sitting cross-legged with my back straight, closing my eyes, placing my hands palm down on my knees, and then counting each inhale and exhale to the count of ten. When my mind begins to wander, I simply bring my awareness back to my breath and start counting again. This meditation practice helps me see my thought process with crystal clarity. When my mind starts wandering from my breath and my counting process, I instantly stop myself to see whether my mind is caught up in thoughts of doubt and fear or if my thoughts are filled with trust and love. If my thoughts are filled with doubt and fear, I acknowledge these thoughts (without judgment) and their lack of gentleness, and then peacefully let them go.

The more you are able to "catch" your negative thoughts and peacefully let them go, the more your thinking will start to change and the more you will be able to train yourself to do away with self-limiting and self-defeating thought patterns. This transformation has to do with the refocusing of your energy on kindness and love versus judgment and fear.

Once you have been able to catch your negative thoughts, you can then use the power of affirmations to help solidify a new and healthy relationship to your inner dialogue. Affirmations are simply reminders, a gentle nudge to your conscious and subconscious mind that you mean business. These positive affirmations will give you the strength and determination to believe in yourself and your great healing power. They will also center and ground you in trust and love and help you to let go of all fear-based responses. Here is an example of an affirmation written by Louise L. Hay in her book *You Can Heal Your Life*:

> In the infinity of life where I am, all is perfect, whole, and complete. I no longer choose to believe in old limitations and lack. I now choose to begin to see myself as the Universe sees me—perfect, whole, and complete. The truth of my Being is that I was created perfect, whole, and complete. I will always be perfect, whole, and complete. I now choose to live my life from this understanding. I am in the right place at the right time, doing the right thing. All is well in my world.

As you are able to continue to nurture and refine your thought process through the practice of regular meditation and the use of healing affirmations, you will gradually transform your beliefs into powerful and supportive guides for your journey of self-healing. Through this up-lifted presence, you will easily be able to relax and calm your mind, dissipate all unnecessary stress, and allow a great healing energy to flow throughout your life.

Exercise: The Inner Dialogue

Your inner dialogue is directly connected to the way in which you perceive yourself. By paying close attention to the way you "talk" to yourself, you can begin to transform the way in which you live your life.

The more you catch yourself thinking negative and self-limiting thoughts, the more your thinking will start to change. As I mentioned earlier, your negative thoughts are like weeds that clutter your mind. This next practice serves as a way of weeding out these thoughts and then planting the seeds of positive and loving thoughts.

As in the previous exercise, this exercise should also be done in a quiet place where you will not be disturbed. Before you start, you will need to get a piece of paper or a journal and a pen or pencil.

I would like for you to sit on the floor with a cushion. If this is not possible, sitting in a chair will also work, as will lying down. If you do decide to sit, it is important that you sit with a posture that is straight and firm, but also relaxed—you don't want to be too rigid or tense. If you are lying down, make sure that your body is fully relaxed. You can begin to relax yourself by taking a few deep breaths.

Once you have found a relaxed posture, begin by closing your eyes and focusing your attention on the inward and outward flow of your breath. Do not try and manipulate your breath in any way; simply pay attention to it.

As you are paying attention to your breath, many thoughts will arise. When you are confronted with harsh, judgmental, self-limiting, and negative thoughts, make a mental note of them, and then continue focusing on the flow of your breath. Continue paying attention to your breath and your thought patterns for about ten to fifteen minutes.

After you are finished, write down a few of the overriding negative thought patterns that you observed. If you didn't observe any, you can proceed to the last paragraph of this exercise to practice the healing visualization. If you did, then say each one of the negative thoughts out loud, one at a time, while you repeat these words with it: "I am not (whatever it is you wrote down). I am only Pure Unconditional Love. I am perfect just as I am. I fully accept and trust myself and allow myself to completely let go of this false idea that I am (whatever it is you wrote down). I am only Pure Unconditional Love."

For example, if one of the negative thoughts you wrote was "I feel that I am sick," you would then state: "I am not sick. I am only Pure Unconditional Love. I am perfect just as I am. I fully accept and trust myself and allow myself to completely let go of this false idea that I am sick. I am only Pure Unconditional Love."

Repeat this healing affirmation until you have gone through each of the thoughts that you wrote down. After you have finished repeating each thought with the healing affirmation, I would like you to spend at least five more minutes sitting quietly in meditation. During this five minutes, I would like for you to further allow yourself to feel this feeling of pure unconditional love by thinking of a moment in your life when you felt completely peaceful and content within yourself. Nurturing this feeling within yourself is best achieved by imagining exactly where you were and what was happening at that moment. By mentally re-creating this scene, your mind and your body will start to feel it again. Embracing this feeling will help you to remember that you always have the power to choose to feel good about yourself and your life.

The Message of this Gateway:
What You Perceive is What You Receive

You always have the choice of how you respond to your life. Your responses shape and mold your entire destiny. Your responses are supported by the way in which you perceive things. If you choose to perceive the universe and yourself as good, you will receive this goodness. If you choose to perceive the universe as a place of infinite healing and love, you will receive this abundance of healing and love.

When you rid yourself of all doubt and hesitation, all fear and negativity, you will discover a trust in yourself and in life that will forever sustain you. This trust removes all of your false beliefs that block your ability to be free. You only experience true freedom when you remove these blocks and open yourself to receive the great blessing stored within yourself and within all of life.

Transformation

Life's greatest lesson
is to learn to trust the darkness.
Within the darkness lies the light.
Within the darkness lies the truth.
Within the darkness lies your
soul's true purpose.

After you have come to a full acceptance of suffering and the life process and have developed an unfaltering sense of trust in yourself and in life, you are then able to welcome the most difficult yet most sustaining experience of all—the *experience* of your suffering. Whereas at the first gateway you learn to accept your suffering, at the third gateway you learn how to work with this suffering. By working with your suffering, you learn the wondrous art of transforming all your hardships into opportunities. Again in Victor Frankl's words, "For then what matters is to bear witness to the uniquely human potential at its best, which is to transform a personal tragedy into a triumph, to turn one's predicament into a human achievement."

Only by working through your suffering and venturing into your inner darkness can you transform yourself. Transformation takes place when you embrace the darkness and allow it to bless your life with its regenerative and restorative power.

Darkness is the source of all life. All seeds germinate in darkness. We are all born in the darkness of the womb. Everything in life is supported through this all-pervasive darkness. At some point in our lives, we have come to fear this darkness—a fear that does not allow intimacy with life. It cuts us off from the source of our being. And once this happens, we continually search outside of ourselves for this connection. We live our lives believing that we can find happiness and contentment in material pleasures. We hide, escape, entertain, distract, and continually evade the one thing that will make us truly content—our pain.

Pain, hardship, struggle, and heartache are the fuel for inner transformation. Every great person throughout history has only become great because they endured a very challenging hardship and turned it into an incredible opportunity. Every great musician has journeyed into their own heartache to write the most touching and enduring love songs. Every great writer has gone to the depths of their personal suffering to communicate deep and enduring truths. Every great scientist has been able to delve into the pain and loneliness of the human condition to explore and discover the great mysteries of life on this planet.

In the words of Master Eckhart, the fourteenth-century philosopher and mystic: "Truly, it is in the darkness that one finds the light, so when we are in sorrow, then this light is nearest of all to us." And in the words of the great thirteenth-century poet Rumi, in his poem entitled *Shadow and Light Source Both*, "No matter how fast you run, your shadow keeps up ... But that shadow has been serving you. What hurts you, blesses you. Darkness is your candle. Your limitations are your quest."

The "limitations" that you need to overcome are the hesitancy and unwillingness to embrace your emotions. Your emotions are the keys that unlock the mystery of your suffering and welcome a holy transformation into your life. This transformation is always the journey from separation and fear back into wholeness and love.

In the words of the renowned psychologist Carl Jung, "Emotion is the chief source of all becoming-conscious. There can be no transforming of darkness into light and of apathy into movement without emotion." When you engage with your emotions, you allow your body and mind to heal. Your emotions have the power to renew every part of you. This is because your emotions reveal you to yourself. At any given moment, they show you where you are stuck, how open you are, and to what extent you are embracing the blessing of the present moment and your life. By listening to and embracing the power of your emotions, you allow yourself to be sparked with the raw energy of conscious awareness that will undoubtedly fuel your journey of spiritual transformation.

In order to be healed and given new life and transform life's challenges into the means for a spiritual awakening, you must journey into the abyss where you confront your emotions. The abyss is the world of the subconscious—the part of your brain that organizes your memory, processes your experiences, and stores your emotional pain.

The subconscious makes up more than 98 percent of your mind's activity, so making contact with it by tapping into the deep-seated emotions that lie beneath the surface of your conscious awareness is very important. Once you make contact with these emotions by willingly venturing inwards into your pain and suffering, you witness how you have been cutting yourself off from your heart. The journey into the abyss is actually the journey back into your heart. Only by venturing into this darkness you can release the hidden emotions that have blocked your connection to your heart.

Your emotional life is the heartbeat of your spiritual life. If your emotions are blocked or stagnant, your spiritual life will be stagnant as well. This is a key point in understanding the importance of your connection to your emotions. In my experience, there are two different kinds of emotions. There are either free-flowing emotions or stagnant and stuck emotions. The most common stagnant emotions are resentment, depression, anxiety, and guilt. I label these emotions "stagnant" because they are hiding what you are actually feeling. They act as a façade. They hide and actually stop the flow of what you are truly feeling and eventually leave you lifeless and empty. Stagnant emotions occur after years and years of denying and not expressing how you feel. Eventually unexpressed anger turns into resentment, unexpressed sadness turns into depression, unexpressed fear turns into anxiety, and unexpressed shame turns into guilt.

Oftentimes stagnant emotions occur because of an experience of trauma that happened at some point in our lives. As I briefly mentioned in the Trust chapter, this experience of trauma can lay the foundation of a deep-seated emotional dysfunction and consequent avoidance behaviors. Because of our experience of trauma, we do everything we can to shield ourselves from any type of emotional discomfort that even slightly resembles the pain we experienced. The *American Heritage Dictionary* defines trauma as an emotional shock that causes lasting psychological damage. This "psychological damage" often expresses itself as an inability to deal with the many challenges that life is always presenting. Because of the "emotional shock" of what happened to us, we no longer trust life and because we no longer trust life, we simply shut ourselves down. When we shut ourselves down, we become so void of emotions that our spirit and zest for life severely diminishes.

Our emotions are the blood that flows through the veins of our spiritual body. If our emotions become stagnant, blocked, or cut off, we become spiritually dead. It is through our sadness, our anger, our hurt, our fear that we learn and grow and feel what it is to be truly alive. It is only through engaging with our emotions that we fully embrace our lives. Unfortunately, most of our energy is focused on doing everything we can to avoid any kind of emotional discomfort. Again in Pema Chodron's words:

The sad part is that all we're trying to do is not feel that underlying uneasiness. The sadder part is that we proceed in such a way that the uneasiness only gets worse. The message here is that the only way to ease our pain is to experience it fully. Learn to stay. Learn to stay with uneasiness, learn to stay with the tightening … so that the habitual chain reaction doesn't continue to rule our lives, and the patterns that we consider unhelpful don't keep getting stronger as the days and months and years go by.

In order to fully open yourself to your emotional process you must (1) realize how and where you are stuck, (2) learn to stay with how you are feeling, and (3) let go and forgive. This process takes a tremendous amount of self-awareness. This self-awareness is gained by no longer identifying with your past trauma so that you can learn how to look at yourself objectively. One of the hardest things to do when confronted with trauma is to learn how to stop identifying with it. The experience of trauma sets you up to repeat unconscious behaviors that perpetuate feeling trapped and victimized. This toxic attitude keeps you stuck in an ongoing cycle of fear and continual struggle that does not allow personal healing or transformation to unfold.

Once you face your trauma by sitting with the pain, looking your fear straight in the eye, and accepting and trusting that this experience is what is necessary for you to heal and transform yourself, you soon find your way back into a renewed passion and excitement for life.

As you learn to pierce the pain straight on and use it as fuel for becoming more alive, you gradually re-enter the sacred sanctuary of your soul. Peter Levine, expert on trauma and the healing process, states: "The process of healing trauma can drop us into virtual birth canals of consciousness. From these vantage points, we can position ourselves to be propelled fully into the stream of life. Healing from trauma can be that final instinctive push, that inner shaking and trembling, 'the kick,' that can awaken us and lead us on a journey home."

The next two sections will focus on leading you on this "journey home." Your home is the land of your heart. Your journey back into this holy land will lead you into the healing space where all transformation takes place. On this healing journey you will find your way into the most transformative experience of all—forgiveness.

Working Through Pain

The first and second gateway provide you with an openness and gentleness that makes entering the third gateway possible. But what is necessary to enter the third gateway is a willingness—a willingness to fully look at and examine yourself. Openness and gentleness provide the framework for you to feel comfortable and secure enough to relax within your inner world. Within your inner world is where you make the decision to transform your pain into strength, your heartache into wisdom, your sorrow into joy.

IF YOU WANT
To grow
Then you need
To cry
And let go
And feel
Your own soul
And heal
Your own heart
And embrace
Your own pain
And slow down
Enough
To open yourself
To love
And make peace
With who you are
And all that you
Have been through
Resting quietly
In the perfect stillness
Of each and every one
Of your life experiences

The work of examining your inner world is the work of alchemy. This alchemy happens when you take the raw material of your life and purify it with the conviction and steadfastness of your heart. This process takes the heaviness of your pain and hurt and turns it into the gold of your forgiveness and love. Once your heart becomes purified through constant attention to your emotions, you become ready to transform yourself. By embracing your emotions, you allow your pain to soften, which instantly makes way for new growth. Again in the words of the poet Rumi: "Every midwife knows that not until a mother's womb softens from the pain of labor will a way unfold and the infant find that opening to be born. Oh friend! There is a treasure in your heart. It is heavy with child. Listen. All the awakened ones, like trusted midwives, are saying, welcome this pain, it opens the dark passage of grace."

Welcoming your pain begins once you realize how and where you are stuck. In my experience, being stuck has always been associated with the many defense mechanisms that tried to distract me from dealing with my life. These defense mechanisms usually reveal themselves as an apathy and indifference toward life. The first step toward healing yourself is to learn how to break apart apathy and indifference—which means recognizing and understanding your comfort zones. As I mentioned in the Acceptance chapter, it is your comfort zones that keep your suffering at bay. It is your comfort zones that stop you from welcoming "the dark passage of grace." You can begin your healing process by watching how you distract yourself when you feel any kind of emotional discomfort. Do you go shopping? Do you watch too much TV or spend too much time on the Internet? Do you spend your time obsessively worrying about insignificant details? Begin by paying attention to how you spend your time. This will reveal to you how you avoid and defend yourself from living an authentic and meaningful life.

Perhaps one of the most unhealthy things we can do is repress and block our emotions. For inner growth and transformation to take place, we need to allow our energy to move and flow. If our emotions become stuck because of our need to stay comfortable and safe, there is no possible way to heal ourselves. The only way to keep our energy moving and foster the healing process is to allow our emotions to be fully expressed and released. All of our emotions are important, even our negative ones. What is important is that we are honest with ourselves about these emotions and that we learn to use these emotions to gain further self-awareness. In the words of Candace Pert, an internationally acclaimed research professor and expert on the emotions and the healing process, author of *Molecules of Emotion*:

> Let me begin to answer by saying that I believe all emotions are healthy, because emotions are what unite the mind and body. Anger, fear, and sadness, the so-called negative emotions, are as healthy as peace, courage, and joy. To repress these emotions and not let them flow freely is to set up a dis-integrity in the system, causing it

to act at cross-purposes rather than a unified whole. The stress this creates, which takes the form of blockages and insufficient flow of peptide signals to maintain function at the cellular level, is what sets up the weakened conditions that can lead to disease. All honest emotions are positive emotions.

In order to allow our emotions to flow freely, we must learn how to respond to them appropriately. When we react to our emotions by being too defensive, passive, or aggressive, we instantly take away the opportunity to embrace what our emotions are trying to communicate. Reacting to our emotions can often happen very quickly and many times leaves us wondering why we acted so foolishly and carelessly. When we haven't dealt with our emotional lives, it can be very easy to lash out at others with our anger and frustration. The way that we tend to express ourselves externally in the world is directly related to the way we feel about ourselves. So, if we do not feel good about ourselves, we wind up causing others harm. This abusive cycle is the root of so much of the suffering in the world.

Instead of quickly reacting to our emotions out of anger and frustration, we can learn to patiently (and slowly) respond with a curiosity and inquisitiveness. The way that I have learned (and am still learning) to not react to my emotions and instead remain curious and inquisitive about them is to do my best to view them like an old friend that I never quite got along with, coming to visit me over and over again. The message of this friend is to always listen, listen, listen. When I listen to my emotions instead of quickly reacting to them, I can actually hear what message they have for me. Once I listen long enough, I can begin to make peace with this old friend and eventually learn to let go of our age-old struggle. I love this Rumi poem entitled "The Guest House," which further illustrates this idea.

This being human is a guest house.
Every morning a new arrival.

A joy, a depression, a meanness,
some momentary awareness comes
as an unexpected visitor.

Welcome and entertain them all!
Even if they're a crowd of sorrows,
who violently sweep your house
empty of its furniture,
still, treat each guest honorably.
He may be clearing you out
for some new delight.

The dark thought, the shame, the malice,
meet them at the door laughing,
and invite them in.

Be grateful for whoever comes,
because each has been sent
as a guide from beyond.

Once you see begin to see how and where it is you get stuck, you can then learn to sit with and befriend how you truly feel. Instead of running, hiding, and escaping, you can allow yourself the freedom to peacefully and comfortably sit down and get to know what message your emotions have for you. This takes a willingness to want to explore how you feel. I believe there is no better way to experience your emotions than that of crying. For me, it has always been an experience of crying that has helped me move through a stagnant or blocked period of my life. Crying is an instant and immediate cure for breaking apart apathy and allowing healing energy to flow again. Crying allows you to be vulnerable. It allows blocked feelings to be exposed, which instantly brings a warmth and a light back into all the cold and dark places within your inner landscape. Crying reflects your willingness to allow life to touch you. It also allows you to experience your brokenness, your broken heart, which is essential for new growth and healing to begin. Crying is your message to life that you are ready to let go and open yourself to what it is trying to reveal to you and through you.

After four months of chemotherapy, I had experienced so much pain and discomfort that I had developed a "toughness" that I thought was necessary for me to deal with the overwhelming challenge and difficulty of my situation. I thought that, as a man, I was supposed to "toughen up" and not allow myself to break down and cry. Like most men, I thought crying showed weakness.

I can remember seeing my father cry only about two or three times in my whole life. It just seemed like something I wasn't supposed to do. Even when faced with one of the hardest situations in my life, for the most part, I remained unwilling to experience the healing release of emotion.

During the last week of this four-month period of chemotherapy sessions, I attended a Ziggy Marley concert. Ziggy Marley, the son of the legendary reggae musician Bob Marley, exudes the same positive message as his father, which is for everybody to come together with music and be healed through the divine presence of love.

Because of my love for reggae music, I went to the concert even though I was probably too sick to attend. I stood in the front row so I could hold onto the gate when I felt too tired to stand. I remember feeling like every song was being sung for me. I cried my way through the concert. Ziggy sang about finding mercy in every sunrise and being reborn every night—noting that there is always a rainbow in the sky if you look for it. In another song, Ziggy states that no matter how many questions you ask, the truth never changes—and you have to deal with it.

After two hours of his uplifting songs and his poignant message, he had everybody in the concert form a huge circle around the auditorium and then hold hands and pray for peace. During the prayer circle, I realized how isolated I had felt in my life. I realized how unwilling I had been to open myself to receive life. I had shut myself down because of my fear and pain. While looking at the hundreds of loving faces surrounding me, I felt a strong desire and longing to be connected. I had felt disconnected for so long. While holding hands and praying, I began to cry some more. I felt the love and peace fill the auditorium and it overwhelmed me. It instantly brought me into a space of connectedness and healing. I was overwhelmed with emotion. I hadn't felt that much in a very long time. I felt renewed and uplifted, inspired and transformed.

This renewed connection helped support my future growth into transformation and healing. I gradually learned to stay connected to my inner world with all the uncomfortable, prickly, and thorny emotions that continually arise by always asking myself this question: "Do I want to feel connected to my life and live my life to the fullest or do I want to feel disconnected and live my life half asleep?" My answer has always been to live my life to the fullest, which means attending to and fully experiencing every emotion. This means that I don't block and repress my emotions with an unhealthy need to feel numb and disinterested. Instead, I allow my emotions to flow freely.

Opening yourself to your inner world of your emotions means that you will be pushed to your limit. Your emotions will teach you what you are most hesitant to learn. They will guide you to places you are most reluctant to be. They will challenge you when you'd rather be

TRULY LIVE
By allowing yourself
To forgive
Letting go
Of everything
That has held you back
Putting to rest
Anything that has forced
You to see lack
Instead of wholeness
For now it is time
To take back
With a forgiveness
That heals
With a forgiveness
That unpeels
All the thick layers
Of hurt
To reveal your soul
Bringing you back together
With a restorative power
That makes you whole

left alone. This is the work that is required for personal transformation. As the great philosopher Socrates once said, "The unexamined life is not worth living."

Forgiveness

The message of every pain and sorrow is to forgive. The message of every dis-ease is to forgive. The message of every broken heart is to forgive. Forgiveness is the medicine that you feed to your pain. Once you nourish your pain with forgiveness, you begin to make your return journey from fear back to love. In the words of the great Martin Luther King, Jr., "He who is devoid of the power to forgive, is devoid of the power to love." Forgiveness is your declaration of love in the face of fear. It is your flag of surrender that you wave in the face of suffering.

Once you have made intimate contact with your hurt and pain, it then becomes time to forgive. It is within the realm of forgiveness that the abyss opens up, transforms every part of your past, and grants you new life. The power of forgiveness is what cleanses the wounds of your past. When you forgive, you allow the old parts of yourself to be renewed. Once you release your old ways of relating to people and things and especially to yourself, you allow new perspectives to be brought forth. These new perspectives refresh your mind, renew your body, and strengthen your spirit.

In the last section I briefly mentioned the alchemy of turning your pain into strength, your sorrow into joy,

your heartache into wisdom. This alchemy, or transformation, happens through a purification process. For
this transformation to unfold, you must first learn to
willingly embrace your emotional pain. After you embrace your pain, you then must purify it with the tonic
of forgiveness. Forgiveness is the power that turns your
pain into strength, your sorrow into joy, your heartache
into wisdom.

What makes the act of forgiveness so challenging is
the very easy tendency to react to emotional pain instead
of embracing it. Reacting to our pain takes away the ability to be empowered and immediately throws away the
opportunity to use this pain to transform ourselves.

The only way for your hurt to transform itself is for
you to give it understanding and gentleness. Without a
space for it to breathe—to feel wanted and accepted—it
cannot release itself.

After all my cancer treatments were finished, I knew
that what I most needed to do was forgive. I knew that
this was not going to be easy to do, because trauma lin-
gers in our memories and we habitually react to our
emotions, but that it was necessary in order for me to
truly heal. For me, this meant revisiting the place where
the pain began.

The trauma I experienced at age fourteen included
a difficult surgery, a long delay of puberty, being told I
would always be infertile, the messy divorce of my parents, and the normal challenges of every fourteen-year-
old. I spent the ages of fourteen through eighteen in Key

West, Florida. I knew that in order to begin to forgive, I would have to journey back there.

While I was back in Key West, I visited all my old haunts including my old house, my old high school, the White Street pier where I sat and watched the ocean for hours, the streets where I delivered newspapers, the restaurants where I hung out with my friends, and the doctors' offices where I went to get my monthly check-ups and shots.

While exploring the old streets of my past, I could recall a lot of trauma, but noted there was also a lot of joy. Not everything was as bad as I had remembered. As soon as I opened the gate to my old house on Grinnell Street and looked into my old bedroom window, I actually felt a sense of excitement. After I looked into the window, I sat on the steps and reminisced.

As I was sitting on my old porch, I was quickly brought back in time. I felt as if I was waiting for my fourteen-year-old self to come back from school and walk into the house, put on the video game system, and get a soda from the fridge. I could see myself so clearly that I forgot for a while that I was even sitting there reminiscing.

What moved me the most was not my trauma and de-spair, but actually my confidence and poise. As I looked back into time, I could see myself as quite an extraordi-nary young man. There I was, getting on my bicycle and taking myself to my doctor's appointments to get testos-terone shots, working two jobs, and going to school and taking college courses. I could see myself talking to my mother and father and telling them that everything was going to work out just fine.

After beginning to realize that I was not as helpless as I had thought, I began to question where my extreme resistance to this time in my life had come from. A stream of questions began to fill my mind. "What was it that made me stop believing in myself? When did I lose my self-confidence and poise? How did my inner strength turn into insecurity? When did I close myself off to life?"

As I began to explore these questions, I got an image of myself in college getting intoxicated. I began to see myself as a nineteen-year-old trying so hard to fit in. Because of the numerous insecurities I had due to the trauma of my surgery, I had become completely unsure of myself. Since my sexuality was extremely wounded, I felt awkward around almost everyone. In my desperate need to be perceived as "normal," I compromised myself tremendously. By compromising myself for the sake of making friends and meeting girls, I traded in my authenticity for insecurity. Instead of being comfortable with who I was, I started being someone I wasn't. It was right here where I realized how all my troubles began and then my entire past all started to make sense.

By revisiting these places of my past, I was able to befriend and love them because, for the first time in my life, I was able to understand them. By seeing into my past with this understanding and insight, I was finally able to let go and forgive.

In the words of the Buddha, "To understand every-thing is to forgive everything." When you understand everyone and everything, you empower yourself to break down the barriers that stand in your way of let-ting go and moving on. These barriers are the suffocat-ing emotional reactions such as resentment, depres-sion, anxiety, and guilt that block your true feelings and do not allow the freedom to heal. Once you are able to carefully examine these barriers, you begin to see how you are cutting yourself off from living your own life. These barriers force an unhealthy way of engaging with every aspect of your life. They force you to disconnect from yourself, people, and life's experiences with ongo-ing judgment, harshness, and criticism. With under-standing, you will be able to break down these barriers and reconnect with yourself and with everything else. With understanding, you will be able to harness your self-awareness to see why and how you and others get stuck in fear instead of empowered through love. With this continued understanding, you will be able to let go and forgive. This power of forgiveness will heal every part of your life.

How to Enter this Gateway: Open Your Heart

At the third gateway, you enter into the brilliant land-scape of your inner world—your heart. Your heart-space contains your inner wisdom. It contains your power. It is the only place where you are able to fully transform yourself. In the words of the Talmud, "Your heart will give you greater counsel than all the world's scholars."

The main practice of connecting with and opening the heart is done through art. Art is the alchemy of purifying and softening the heart. The practice of creating art acts as a direct passageway into your subconscious mind—the mysterious inner landscape of images, symbols, dreams, and emotions. By exploring these inner realms, you expose the hidden parts of yourself that need healing. Art allows you to open your heart. Again in the words of the poet Rainer Maria Rilke:

> Everything is gestation and bringing forth. To let each impression and each germ of a feeling come to completion wholly in itself, in the dark, in the inexpressible, the unconscious, beyond the reach of one's own intelligence, and await with deep humility and patience the birth-hour of a new clarity: that alone is living the artist's life.

By engaging with the artistic process, you learn how to transform your emotions into something beautiful and divine. This process allows you to gain new perspectives and new ways of seeing things. It also creates an opening in your mind for increased objectivity. Instead of becoming stuck within a specific emotional state, you skillfully learn how to work with whatever emotion you are dealing with to eventually transcend and uplift the experience. The artistic process can be quite exhilarating and transformative. In a sense, you release and give birth to this emotional state through a finished painting, poem, photograph, sculpture, etc. This piece of work then allows you to see into your experience with new eyes. This process allows you the safe and nurturing space you need to grow and heal.

By using your emotions as tools to express and heal the deepest parts of yourself, you develop a life-affirming attitude that is always focused on creating personal meaning. You engage your mind in learning how to see things with new perspectives. You learn to illuminate a healing light over everything that is dark and scary in your inner world. As the always insightful and wise author and speaker Wayne W. Dyer states, "If you change the way you look at things, the things you look at change." This is exactly what the artistic process helps you to achieve.

We all are artists. We all have the capability to create art. It just takes a willingness to work with the raw emotions in your life. Once you decide to explore your suffering, the expression will take care of itself.

I spent many days and nights in a hospital bed without anything to do but just sit there feeling sick and tired. I had so many emotions welling up inside of me and I was barely expressing any of them. On one of my extremely emotional days, I received a package from a friend that included a beautifully decorated journal. Once I opened that journal, I didn't stop writing until I fell to sleep that night. This creative fervor soon became the driving force behind my ability to sustain a stable and relaxed state of mind. Expressing all of my emotions not only helped me process and make sense of how I was feeling, but also helped me become extremely passionate about writing poetry. I began to write day and night—poetry, journal entries—and when not writing I also did sketches and drawings. I can't imagine what the rest of my time in the hospital would have been like without it. Every time I would write a journal entry or write a poem or draw a picture, I would instantly feel lighter, more at peace, and more in touch with my experience.

Here is a poem from my journal that I wrote about my experiences with dealing with a year of cancer treatments:

> Can't believe the last year
> It's been like a hurricane
> Been torn between the love and fear
> Just trying to deal with the pain
> I have seen the hallow darkness
> Wrestled with my insecurity
> Felt the depths of my sadness
> And breathed in the mystery
>
> The coolness of this winter day
> I feel deep in my bones
> The memories find a way
> To make me feel alone
> When death comes in the night
> There's no way you can hide
> I had to face the haunting sight
> While a part of me died

The full moon in the distance
I watch it and ponder
The silence that is endless
And the dreams that I wonder
The stillness in the landscape
Gives me more than I need
The wisdom of no escape
And the faith to believe

Whenever I write, I use a stream-of-consciousness writing style. This writing style allows me to express everything inside of myself without stopping to think about it, which usually stops my writing flow. Whenever I feel the need to express myself, I simply start writing, without thinking of what I should write about or how I should say it. Whatever images, words, or ideas arise are written down without judgment. This writing style doesn't include the use of punctuation, which also can cause you to slow down and start thinking too much. Oftentimes, I revise the poem or journal entry later on so it makes more sense, but most of the time it is perfect just as it is.

The stream-of-consciousness writing style is based on the philosophy of "First thought, best thought." The late poet Allen Ginsberg coined this phrase to describe using writing to fearlessly break through the conscious mind to deliver and express the absolute truth that usually lies beneath your conscious awareness. When you write whatever surfaces in your mind without second-guessing yourself, you are able to pierce through the many layers of the rational mind, which is always caught up in making judgments and futile comparisons. In the words of Natalie Goldberg, author of *Writing Down the Bones:* "First thoughts have tremendous energy. The internal censor usually squelches them, so we live in the realm of second and third thoughts, thoughts on thought, twice and three times removed from the direct connection of the first fresh flash." The absolute truth is achieved by making contact with the "first fresh flash" of the subconscious, which is beyond judgments and beyond the surface-level thoughts of the conscious mind. Once you make contact with the subconscious, as I described earlier on in the chapter, you will be able to unleash the great power stored inside of yourself. This is because your subconscious holds the key to unlock the many closed doors that have kept you isolated from yourself. Once this door to yourself is opened, you instantly release all the outdated emotional patterns that have been stuck inside of you and causing so many disturbances. Once these are cleared out, you are free to live without the heaviness of sorrow and the unnecessary burden of guilt and shame. Here is an example of a stream of consciousness that I wrote after I returned from my trip to Paris that I mentioned in the introduction. The Paris trip was the culmination of my healing process, marking my transformation from a "cancer patient" into a healthy and whole new person:

Over the great ocean into another land into an ancient
city filled with brilliant cathedrals built in eternity with
infinite devotion forcing me to my knees bringing my
soul to tears in the immensity of beauty that filled each
molecule of air with light that filled each pore of flesh
with awe and I began to drown in this sea of inspiration
as I walked along the river over the romantic bridges
next to majestic castles all illumined by lights arising like
a great song in majestic harmonies played one after the
other instantly filling me with more and more light and
all I could do was dance with this light and give birth to
an ancient muse in a language of stars and I got so completely drunk with every new image—so drunk that my
legs could not move and so dizzy from the overwhelming sensation of birth that death no longer made any
sense to me and as I continued to walk through the poetry of these cobblestone streets consumed with flowers and sculptures and gorgeous desires I let go of the
old decaying self inside of me realizing that with light
I could sculpt anything and so I transformed this dark
past filled with broken images of sickness and age old
doubt and turned it into the holy images of this ancient
timeless city that crowned me king of life and love giving me new eyes and new thoughts and a new vision
that will forever guide and sustain me

The use of writing and artistic expression is an incredible tool for inner transformation. Many research studies
have documented how releasing one's emotions substan-
tially helps boost the immune system. When emotions
flow freely and openly, the alchemy of self-transformation is allowed to unfold. The wonderful book *A Course*

In Miracles states, "Miracles are everyone's right, but purification is necessary first." This purification is the work of beholding and embracing each and every emotion and allowing them to open you to the deep wisdom of yourself. The miracle is that you are able to transform your fear into love, your hurt into forgiveness, your sorrow into joy.

Exercise: On Hurt and Forgiveness

Entering your inner world of darkness is the most challenging experience on your healing journey. It instantly pushes you beyond your limitations and breaks you open into a vulnerability that allows new growth to take place. This new growth can only happen when you make the decision to face the inner hurt that you have been holding on to. Healing unfolds when you consciously release this burden. The only way this burden can be released is through the release of your emotions. This next exercise allows you to first recognize what burdens you are holding on to and then to consciously release them.

For this exercise you will need to have a couple pieces of paper or a journal and a pen or pencil to write with. Sit down in a quiet room where you will not be disturbed. First, I would like you to close your eyes and place both of your hands over your heart. Allow yourself to patiently feel what hurt is stored inside of you. Begin by examining your hurt by asking your hurt these questions: "Where do you come from? What do you look like? What is your message for me? Why can I not let you go?" Sit with these questions until your emotional hurt rises to the surface of your conscious awareness. Once it arises, I would like you to experience your hurt to the full by allowing yourself to cry. Crying is the best way to dislodge this emotion and allow it to release itself. Crying instantly tells your hurt that you are not afraid of it.

Once you have allowed yourself to release your emotion, I would like for you to remove your hands from your heart and instead move them to your shoulders so that you are hugging yourself. (Your right hand should be grasping your left shoulder and your left hand grasping your right shoulder.) Next, state this affirmation: "I accept my hurt. I accept my life experiences. I accept myself." State this affirmation as many times as necessary for you to feel that you are fully embracing and befriending yourself and your hurt.

Secondly, I would like for you to write down on a piece of paper these three sentences—leaving enough room in between each sentence for you to elaborate upon them. These sentences are: "I forgive myself for _____," "I forgive life for _____," and "I forgive (whomever people they may be) for _____."

For example, when I did this exercise, the sentence "I forgive myself" went like this: "I forgive myself for the hurt that I have caused to others. My intention was to never cause harm. I was wounded. I myself was hurt. At the time I was not capable of being gentle with you or the situation. My anger was my reaction to my unresolved hurt. This hurt was the reason I took it out on you. This hurt was the reason I made the mistake of blaming and accusing you. I am sorry for causing this hurt. I fully forgive myself."

After you state each of these three or more statements, I would like for you to sit quietly for at least five more minutes, allowing yourself to fully embrace the feeling of forgiveness inside of you.

The Message of this Gateway: Turn Your Pain into Power

By connecting with what is inside your heart, you open yourself to the great power stored inside. By working with this raw energy, you create a strong and willful intention to transform all of your struggles into power. It is important to remember that all power comes from the heart, all wisdom comes from the heart, all strength comes from the heart.

As you work through your pain and make intimate contact with your emotions, your whole life will become transformed. Your emotions are your greatest teachers and when you embrace them, you instantly receive their life-changing lessons. This intimacy with your emotions will help you to become fearlessly self-aware. This self-awareness will transform your life into an endless opportunity for healing and transformation.

PERSONAL POWER

WHEN YOU LET GO
of resistance,
you experience truth.
When you embrace truth,
you experience presence.
When you live within this presence,
you are instantly healed.

Once your heart has been awakened by consciously working through your pain and transforming each and every life circumstance into an opportunity for empowerment and growth, you quickly find your way into the fourth gateway. Since your heart has now been awakened, you are brought to the essence and meaning of the spiritual path—compassion.

Compassion is the direct result of having embraced your suffering (rather than stagnantly wallowing in it) and turning it into something of great value and meaning. Think of the many great people throughout the last century who have used their suffering for a greater cause. To name just a few: Martin Luther King, Jr., Gandhi, Victor Frankl, Nelson Mandela, the Dalai Lama, Thich Nhat Hanh, and Elie Wiesel. They learned how to transform suffering into an opportunity to awaken their hearts and the hearts of humanity—and you also have the power to do so.

Personal power lies within the ability to nurture your compassion by sharing the many lessons you have learned in your life to help others on their own journey through life. The more you help, the stronger your compassion becomes, and the more personal power you develop.

The more challenging and difficult your experiences are the more passion and inner conviction you will feel to help others. I recently read the extraordinary book, *Left to Tell,* which describes Immaculée Ilibagiza's amazing story of surviving the Rwandan holocaust. The horrors she experienced were unbearable. She witnessed the colossal atrocity of almost all of her family and friends, neighbors, teachers, and townspeople all being brutally exterminated. She witnessed her entire country being overtaken by hatred, violence, and fear, yet this amazingly inspired woman found it in herself to overcome this suffering by focusing all her energy on God. When faced with the man that was responsible for killing her mother and brother, she simply said, "I forgive you." Through her tremendous fearlessness and courage, she was not only able to gracefully endure the suffering that she witnessed, but was also able to turn the experience of her hardship into something to benefit the world. After the holocaust ended, she began working for the United Nations and, quickly after that, she established a foundation to help others heal from the debilitating effects of genocide and war. In her own eloquent words:

> I saw the circle of hatred and mistrust forming in those innocent eyes, and I knew that God was showing me another reason. He'd spared me. I vowed that one day, when I was strong and capable enough, I would do everything I could to help the children orphaned by genocide. I

would try to bring hope and happiness to their lives, and to steer them away from embracing the hatred that had robbed them of their parents, and of a family's love.

Stephen Hawking is another great example of an individual that has used his own "personal tragedy" and turned it into a "triumph," for the benefit of helping the world. Even though he has suffered from ALS (amyotrophic lateral sclerosis) and has been confined to a wheelchair for almost forty-five years, Hawking has made some of the greatest scientific discoveries of our lifetime. He found it in himself to accept his situation, trust and believe in himself, and gracefully use his very challenging situation as an opportunity to better himself. By furthering himself in this way, he has not only extended his life by many, many years, but also has been able to see beyond his own predicament and into a larger perspective of life. In his own life-affirming words, "Before my condition had been diagnosed, I had been very bored with life. There had not seemed to be anything worth doing. But shortly after I came out of hospital, I dreamt that I was going to be executed. I suddenly realized that there were a lot of worthwhile things I could do if I were reprieved.... I would sacrifice my life to save others."

This idea of sacrifice is a key component in how you develop personal power. The fact is, once you learn how to sacrifice your needs for a greater need, you develop the highest form of compassion and personal power that exists. When you give yourself to a purpose that is greater than yourself, such as being a parent, helping another person heal, raising money for people less fortunate than yourself, helping save the environment, or whatever the cause may be, you learn to live life with a wide-open heart. By living with this compassionate presence, your inner light begins to shine very, very brightly and you become extremely capable of not only healing yourself, but also of healing the world. This compassion will fill your life to the brim with heartfelt purpose, passionate direction, and great personal meaning.

Carefully looking at the choices you are making in life is very important. If you decide to make choices that further your sense of purpose and meaning, confidence and inner strength, you are following the right path. This path is the path with a heart. In the words of the very influential author Carlos Castaneda, "Look at every path closely and deliberately. Try it as many times as you think necessary. Then ask yourself and yourself alone one question … Does this path have a heart? If it does, the path is good. If it doesn't, it is of no use." A path with a heart is one that affirms your inner truth, grounds you in your center, and allows you to unfold your precious gifts. This heartfelt path will allow you to use these gifts to help others in the world. At the fourth gateway, you embrace this "path with a heart" by learning how to live from your center and committing yourself to doing what you most love. Once you decide to make these two very important decisions, you will harness your personal power in extraordinary ways.

Doing What You Love

The experience of suffering had me grappling with meaning. I wanted to know why these experiences were happening to me. I wanted to know why I was having to face such darkness. I wanted to know "why me." It wasn't until I stopped asking *why*, though, that I learned *how* to transform my suffering. Our life's purpose is awakened through this very important mental shift. Once again in Viktor Frankl's words, "The way in which a man accepts his fate and all the suffering it entails, the way in which he takes up his cross, gives him ample opportunity—even under the most difficult circumstances—to add a deeper meaning to his life." As I previously mentioned, suffering is nothing more than suffering unless you make the choice to let it open you to your soul—revealing to you how much power you have to turn the opportunity of a lifetime into a miraculous and divine undertaking.

This decision is rooted in your ability to fearlessly look darkness in the eye. Once you are able to do this, you awaken your ability to see. What you see with your renewed and transformed eyes is your passion illuminated both within and without. Your passion is the direct outcome of living your life with a willingness to harness the darkness to illuminate more and more light. This light flows from your ability to nurture your inner world through the experience of more and more love.

The first thing I noticed after I relinquished the struggle to figure out *why* I was suffering and instead focused on *how* to transform it was a renewed feeling of energy and enthusiasm. Instead of wrestling with myself, I began accepting and facing the challenges before me. I started reading stories about people who had courageously overcome many of life's challenges, and was amazed at how empowered they had become through these experiences. Immediately I became passionate about something—I wanted to become one of those people! I wanted to not only heal myself from cancer, but I also wanted to live my life with enthusiasm and passion. I wanted to feel excited about my life. I wanted to feel good about being me. I wanted to feel happy when I looked into the mirror to see myself. I wanted to feel thrilled to greet another day and another opportunity to fully embrace my life.

This passion first revealed itself through the desire to express myself through writing poetry. Being brought up by a mother who majored in English literature and a father who was a librarian and a poet, I had always had an affinity for writing. By giving myself to this gift, I quickly began transforming my suffering, while also adding a renewed spark of passion into my life. This passion helped me realize that I always had the ability to develop personal meaning and renew my energy simply by doing what felt good for me to do.

My father, who recently died of ALS, was faced with one of the most challenging of life's circumstances, yet he still managed to achieve new goals. My father was almost completely paralyzed, only able to move one finger on his right hand. Amazingly, he used this finger to do what he loved, which was to write poetry. Sometimes it would take a very long time to write a poem, but he still stuck with it, because he knew how important it was for his state of mind and his overall well-being. Before he died, he successfully published his book, which now stands as a monumental testimony to the strength of will and the power of one's dreams.

I love Thoreau's famous quote that further illustrates this:

> If one advances confidently in the direction of her dreams, and endeavors to live the life which she has imagined, she will meet with a success unexpected in common hours. She will put some things behind, will pass an invisible boundary; new, universal, and more liberal laws will begin to establish themselves around and within her; old laws will be expanded and interpreted in her favor in a more liberal sense, and she will live with a license of a higher order of beings.

If your time is used nurturing your gifts and talents, it will awaken a major transformation in your life. This transformation unfolds when you decide to live your heart's true path. When you commit yourself to cultivating the gifts you were born with versus the impediments that you have been conditioned with, your life takes on new meaning. Dr. Rachel Naomi Remen, author of the wonderful and inspiring book, *Kitchen Table Wisdom,* describes this process as "…letting go of everything that isn't you—all of the expectations, all of the beliefs—and becoming who you are." She also states, "What we believe about ourselves can hold us hostage."

Removing the chains of expectations and the false limitations about who we should or shouldn't be, what we should or shouldn't be doing, how we should or shouldn't be living takes a tremendous amount of courage. Whether these expectations have come from family, friends, or society doesn't matter—what matters is that we break free from them. The only way to break free from these chains is to do what your heart is compelled to do.

It wasn't until I got sick with cancer that I was able to finally remove these disabling and crippling chains. The intensity of suffering removed everything that wasn't necessary or important in my life. It purified me by confronting me with my own mortality. It continually asked me, "How are you going to spend your limited amount of time in this lifetime? Are you going to spend it enjoying your time, doing what you love, or are you going to waste your time on things that do not matter?"

Once I made the decision to refuse to focus my energy on what I didn't want or need, I gradually began to manifest what it was I truly wanted and needed. As I previously mentioned, what I most wanted was to heal and feel a renewed passion for life. By refocusing my intention on my gift of writing, I not only helped to heal myself, but I also became passionate about so many other things. I started doing yoga and tai chi, meditation and chanting, emotional release work, and healing visualizations and qigong. This renewed passion filled every part of my life—it was contagious. It opened me to the process of healing in a way that I had never experienced before. It allowed me to witness a spiritual presence inside of myself that I had never met. Most importantly, this renewed passion opened the doorway of compassion that has been and continues to be the most powerful and healing force in my life.

After my experiences with cancer, I went on to receive a master's degree in professional counseling, and also became a certified Reiki Master. I became driven and compelled to share my passion of healing. This is also the purpose of my writing practice, which writing this book has helped me fulfill.

It is no accident that the word "compassion" has the word "passion" in it. Once you awaken your passion, you quickly feel the need to share this passion with others, which gives rise to compassion—the experience of boundless kindness and love. This kindness and love is your birthright. It is the source of who and what you are and when you connect to it, you embrace the sacredness of your time with a great power that blesses everyone and everything around you.

Living from Your Center

Right after my last surgery, I had a very powerful dream about connecting with personal power. In the dream, I was standing outside the hospital, looking in the window, watching the doctors operate on me. After a while standing outside, I started feeling that they no longer could operate on me, that I was the only one that knew how to do it. So I tore out the window, jumped into the operating room, and told the doctors to leave. As I looked into my body, I immediately saw the tumor. When I went to cut it out, there was a watch attached to it. When I woke up, I didn't have to spend any time trying to decode the dream's message—I knew exactly what it meant—it meant it was now my time to heal.

For a long time while I was undergoing treatment for cancer, I did not feel that I was the one guiding my healing process. I had given my power away to my doctors because I was so scared. I looked to them for answers to my questions, to give me hope, and to make me feel like I was going to make it through these challenging circumstances. By doing this, I not only became disempowered, but I also was never able to take full responsibility for my healing process. Without this sense of responsibility, it was impossible for me to heal. I was caught in a cycle of fearfully reacting to external events instead of confidently responding from an internal space of poise and centeredness.

This internal connection only arises when you step up to your life to take full responsibility for it. Once you realize that only *you* have the power to create the life you do or do not want, you can begin to face the great responsibility that you behold. However overwhelming this responsibility may seem, it is actually a great relief to know that you always have the power to change your life. Again in the inspiring words of Don Miguel Ruiz, "Your life is the manifestation of your dream; it is an art. And you can change your life anytime if you aren't enjoying the dream. Dream masters create a masterpiece of life; they control the dream by making choices."

Your choices either come from fear or they come from love. Fear-based choices stem from a feeling of needing to control the external world, which forces you to react to events because you do not feel in control of your life, and thus feel a desperate need to find that control. Love-based responses come from a feeling of accepting and trusting that you are always being taken care of and guided, and thus feel that you can relax and peacefully let go into the process of life.

All love-based responses are nurtured from connecting and living from your center. Your center is your place of power where, no matter where you are or what you are doing, you feel and know the truth inside. On a universal level, your truth is that you are a perfect creation of Spirit that is always receiving the healing and renewing emanation of divine love. On a personal level, your truth is unique to you. This truth is revealed through your individual gifts and talents. The way to open yourself to your center to receive these truths is

REALIZE YOUR INNER TRUTH

By knowing that
The only authority
On your life is you
And that everything you do
Either supports or denies
Your ability to view
Yourself and your life
In the proper light—
So open your eyes
To your own awakened insight
And realize that you
Are your own physician
That you can heal
Every broken connection
Mend every thought with compassion
And sustain and unify
Your every action

done through the harmonizing of your inner intention with the outer world.

Your intention is the way you communicate your truth to the world. Your intention is the message of your highest self wanting to be known. You make this intention known by speaking, acting, and thinking in a way that upholds this message. When you speak words of truth that resonate with your highest self, you harmonize with this intention. When you act in ways that uphold the integrity of your intention, your truth, and your highest self, you activate this intention. And when you think thoughts of truth that are aligned with your highest self, you continually regenerate yourself with this holy intention.

It takes tremendous willpower to align yourself with your intention. Our minds are like a caged bird, always trying to escape—and our body is like a pleasure-seeking hedonist, always trying to please itself. Our mind and body are rarely centered without the strength of the personal will reining them in and reminding them who they are supposed to serve. The mind and body would rather serve themselves—but their true master is the soul. It is only through the soul that the mind and body do what they are supposed to do, which is allow the healing presence of your intention and your highest self to be brought forth.

The best way to exert this will and discipline with the mind and body is to learn to stay connected to your physical center that lies in your body. In Japan, this center of the body is called the *hara*. Hara is the word that describes the belly. This physical center holds the key to help you to strengthen your will. This is because the belly is the area of the body that defines the way you hold yourself. If you are not connected to your hara, you will be hunched over, which creates a major barrier in developing personal power. Without the right posture, there is no possible way to feel inner strength and confidence. Your posture dictates how open and relaxed you are, how connected you are to your inner truth and your intention, how well you are able to deal with life's changing circumstances, and to this extent it reveals how power-filled you are. The more you are able to refine and openly reflect this posture in your daily life, the more you will be able to live your life with complete presence and power.

Also, this powerful connection to your hara automatically and spontaneously allows you to openly share your power with others, because you naturally feel compassion for yourself, others, and the world. This compassion is available to you because of your courageous stance to meet each and every moment of your life with fearless authenticity. This "courageous stance" that develops from a connection to your hara is made by simply relaxing your shoulders, slightly bending your knees, and gently arching your lower back so that you are standing upright and firm yet completely relaxed and grounded. The more you live your life with this connection to your hara, reflected in both your body and mind, the more love and compassion is able to flow through you. When

I think of the many teachers who have greatly influenced me, I can always remember their good posture and their warm presence. This always made them seem incredibly approachable and caring. I don't think it was necessarily what they had to teach me that affected me as much as their life-affirming presence. This uplifted presence always left a lasting impression on me. In his book entitled *Hara: The Vital Center of Man*, Karlfried Graf Durckheim states, "With hara increasing a person joyously experiences a new closeness to himself and to the world, to people and things, to nature and God."

The more intimate and self-aware you become within your own being (through the connection to your center), the more capable you are of embracing and generating this healing energy of love and compassion. This healing energy flows through you because of your continual commitment to witnessing and unfolding your truth. When you remain unmoved in this presence of truth, through your deep connection to yourself and the world, you naturally unleash personal power.

How to Enter this Gateway: Nurture Your Truth

The key to opening the fourth gateway, where you learn personal power, is learning how to focus on what you do want versus what you don't want. This power is called the power of intention. Intention allows you to create your world through the passionate activation of your dreams. In Wayne W. Dyer's wonderful book, *The Power of Intention*, he illustrates the amazing power you have when you access this field of intention:

> You must be able to connect to intention, and you can't access and work with intention if you are contemplating the impossibility of being able to intend and manifest ... The Wright Brothers didn't contemplate the staying on the ground of things; Alexander Graham Bell didn't contemplate the non-communication of things; Thomas Edison didn't contemplate the darkness of things. In order to float an idea into your reality, you must be willing to do a somersault into the inconceivable and land on your feet, contemplating what you want instead of what you don't have.

There is a very powerful saying that I have come to live by: "Energy flows where attention goes." Wherever you put your attention in your life is where things will happen. If you put your attention on what you don't have, you will become depressed, and nothing will come your way. However, if you put your attention on what you do have, you will further draw this energy to you, which is what creates an attitude of abundance and prosperity.

Abundance isn't something you have to create—it is already within you and all around you—you simply need to open yourself to receive it. Abundance is witnessed in the beauty and perfection of nature, the beauty and perfection of life, and the beauty and perfection of you! What stops most of us from opening ourselves to receive this abundance is our inability to believe that we deserve it.

The only way that you can open yourself to receive this abundance is to use the power of intention to draw it to you. The more you focus all of your energy on what you want and who you already are, the more these things are drawn to you and the more self-actualized you will become. It's as if you are a magnet and the use of intention is the magnetic field that draws things to you. However, it is important to point out that even if you are not in touch with the power of intention, you are always drawing things to you. Whatever you focus on in your life is what will be drawn to you and what you will ultimately become. If you focus your energy on guilt and shame, you become a guilty person. If you focus your energy on fear and worry, you become an anxious person. If you focus your energy on truth and love, you become a holy person.

Due to the intense trauma that can surround many of life's challenges, you may be impelled to focus your energy and your intention on an unhealthy inner image that inwardly defines and confines you. The inner image that I created for myself was that of a sick and wounded person who wasn't capable of health and wholeness. The supporting storyline that supported this image sounded something like this: "I have cancer. I will always be a sick person. I am not worthy of health. Why should I feel good when I am eventually going to get sick again and die?"

The way I started transforming this inner image about myself was through the use of guided imagery, one of the most powerful tools available for self-healing. Guided imagery helps you to skillfully direct and work with your intention. I started doing different visualizations after all my cancer treatments were over. Even though I was told I was "cancer free," I felt the image of myself as a person that was sick with cancer was still very much alive. I knew that the only way for me to truly heal was to rid myself of this inner image and unhealthy inner dialogue and replace it with a new image and a new dialogue—one of health and vitality. It is important to know that the body immediately responds to whatever image of ourselves we have created. If we have an inner image and belief of ourselves as a sick person, the body eventually becomes sick. If we have the inner image of ourselves as a healthy and radiant person, the body eventually becomes well. Michael Samuel's book *Healing with the Mind's Eye* further illustrates this concept: "When we perceive images as real in the inner world, our body responds to them as if they were real in the outer world … then our immune system's ability to fight infection and destroy cancer cells increases, and our heart rate and blood pressure drop. Somehow the image actually signals each cell. When people imagine that they move their arm, microscopic movements can be detected in the muscles of their arm."

One of the healing visualizations I use consists of the ongoing process of releasing old and stagnant energy and renewing it with vibrant and free-flowing energy, until I feel internally clean and purified. By "clean" and "purified," I mean no longer burdened and poisoned by a toxic and false inner image. This visualization consists of first gently recognizing and acknowledging this unhealthy inner image, next consciously removing it through the power and strength of the will, and lastly replacing it with a new image. For me, recognizing this toxic inner image takes place through entering the first gateway and relaxing my body, which means that I focus on my breathing. I almost always notice that once this toxic inner image arises inside of me, my body and my breath feel tense and stressed. Once I am able to relax my body through deep breathing, I then start to visualize this inner image as dark clumps of tar that are stuck and lodged inside of me. I see this tar as the residue of toxicity that this false inner image has left inside of me. I then imagine grabbing hold of this tar by physically using my hands to grab it and release it. Oftentimes, my hands make aggressive and quick movements to dislodge this energy and eventually purify my energy field. After this toxicity is released, I then imagine a divine image filling me with radiance and light, which instantly makes me feel renewed.

The spiritual practice of intentionally filling yourself with a divine inner image is the cornerstone of all healing and the focus of the rest of this book. By consistently inviting a divine inner image into your being, you gradually start to manifest this energy into your life. By letting go of any and all unhealthy images, you allow yourself to return to the perfection of your divine self. Your divine self knows no false images, faulty words, or unhealthy responses. Your divine self knows only health and wholeness. The healing energy in your life can only be harnessed by connecting yourself to this divine inner image. When you cultivate this divinity within yourself, you instantly nurture your truth. Your truth is that you are a healthy, radiant, and unbelievably powerful person. When you intentionally use your mind, your body, and your spirit to focus on this divine state, you create a space for true healing to occur.

Exercise: Working with Intention

Personal power is the direct outcome of asserting your inner truth. Your inner truth is accessed through the strength of your will. You activate your will through a refocusing of your energy and your attention on your inner divinity instead of the false misconceptions and imposed limitations that do not allow you to empower yourself.

This next exercise will help you to refocus your energy on the things you want to nurture in your life versus the things you don't want. This refocusing of your energy is the passageway into personal power. As for all the exercises, it is good to pick a time of day and a quiet place where you will not be disturbed. This exercise will also require that you have some paper or a journal and a pen or pencil.

The first thing I would like for you to do is make a list of all the barriers that stop you from being empowered. What are the big obstacles and boulders that stop the flow of the river of your life? What are the internal feelings that disrupt your flow? For example, when I did this exercise I wrote: "The things that stop my life from flowing are my continual insecurity—my doubt—my fear of failure—my inability to stay present—my incessant anxiety about my health—my inability to imagine myself empowered."

Secondly, I would like for you to make another list of all the external things that connect you to your bliss and your passion. This list may be some of things that you are currently involved in or things that you would like to be doing but haven't yet. Go ahead and list as many things as you can think of. For example, my list stated: "My bliss and my passion are spiritual practices such as yoga, tai chi, and qigong—I also love to help people with healing work—I love to write—I love to spend time in nature—I love to be with my family—I love to do healing rituals for myself and for others—I love playing music."

Lastly, I would like you to think of three things that you can do to start bridging the gap between these two lists. What are three things you can start doing right now in this very moment to foster this change? What simple actions can you do to refocus your energy? The three things that I wrote were: "I can begin by setting aside at least a half hour a day to do spiritual practice, such as yoga or qigong—I can practice relaxation techniques, such as deep breathing and affirmations at least ten minutes in the morning and ten minutes in the evening to help me dissipate my anxiety and insecurity—and I can begin believing in myself by letting go of my fear of failure by continuing to write and then sending my writing out to different magazines and publishers."

This refocusing of energy takes the strength of your will to keep it going, which means you have to develop an ongoing consistency. Only through consistent effort will these changes take shape in your life. I have witnessed firsthand that, once you make yourself and your passion a priority, you quickly and miraculously transform your life.

The Message of this Gateway: Energy Flows Where Attention Goes

You always have the choice to fill your time with what is most important to you. Connecting with your deepest truth is what will bring true and lasting happiness. By doing what you love, you honor this truth.

As you fearlessly harness the passion that flows from this truth, you connect to the energy of your center. This center allows you to witness and unfold a compassionate presence. When you live from this presence, you are able to attract an abundance of prosperity into your life. This prosperity is reflected in your decision to focus your energy on what is important in your life versus what is not. Once you decide to focus your energy in this way, you will fill your life and the lives of many, many others with an infinite amount of blessings and love.

Spirit

OPEN YOUR MIND
and you become free.
Open your heart
and you become pure.
Open your soul
and you become inspired.

At the fifth gateway, after all the hard work of entering the first four gateways, you receive the greatest blessing there is—the blessing of Spirit. When you stand firm on the earth, even in the midst of great tests and challenges, and feel completely fearless and at one with life, the presence of Spirit awakens in your being. The first four gateways serve as the cleansing and purification that is necessary for the absolutely pure and untainted energy of Spirit to awaken deep within you. Once you have worked through and released all your doubt and insecurity, all your fear and resistance, then your life becomes divinely inspired.

The word *inspiration* means to be in-Spirit. When you are living in-Spirit, you are no longer blinded by a sense of fear that forces you to feel separate from all of creation. A lack of inspiration occurs when you do not feel connected to Spirit. When you are living in-Spirit, though, you witness and see the oneness of creation in every living thing and you feel you are intrinsically part of this beauty. As you feel yourself as part of this amazing beauty, you instantly become overwhelmed with a feeling of awe, wonder, and great respect.

The presence of Spirit provides an invaluable source of energy that is always available to you. This energy exists as pure consciousness—which has infinite potential and is endlessly creative. Everything in the universe has come into being through this energy, which also sustains and nourishes every living thing. The energy in your cells, the energy in the stars, the energy on this earth—all exist as a manifestation of this source. This source is infinitely abundant because it is always creating and manifesting new life. When you connect to this abundance, you nourish yourself with an overflowing power and strength. This abundance is witnessed by connecting with your life force. Your life force exists as a direct manifestation of Spirit. The more you harness your life force, the more Spirit awakens within you.

Your life force can only flow when you have released every blockage that impedes its harmonious and life-renewing power. As I have mentioned in previous chapters, these blockages are all your fear-based ways of responding to life that you must diligently work through in order to restore perfect health to your body, mind, and spirit. The energy of the life force and Spirit exist as the energy of divine love and the only way this energy manifests itself is if there is no fear blocking it. In the book *Healing Yourself the Cosmic Way*, authors Carol K. Anthony and Hanna Moog describe the life force in further detail: "This love, which has been called chi by the Chinese, is our life force. When we are in harmony with the Cosmos, we receive its chi constantly as a renewing force ... Feelings of well-being and of a robust healthiness come from being in a receiving relationship to this abundance of chi energy."

I feel blessed to have had the exhilarating experience of witnessing every blockage in my body and mind dissipate, thereby allowing this divine life force to expand and literally envelop every part of my being. This happened at a Native American healing ceremony in New Mexico. I was invited to go to the healing ceremony right after I found out that the first three rounds of chemotherapy didn't work. Dismayed with Western medicine and looking for more of an experience with my healing process, I decided to go. Even though I had already been through so much with my experiences with cancer, I realized that I hadn't yet really journeyed to the root of what the cancer was trying to communicate with me. Out of my fear and pain, I just wanted the cancer to go away. I didn't want to have to think about it anymore. Approaching the illness in this manner was stopping the cancer from being healed.

During this healing ceremony, I realized how all of my mental and emotional energy was being directed toward resisting the cancer instead of accepting it. I realized that no amount of medicine or surgery was ever going to heal me if I did not make intimate contact with my illness. The cancer was obviously trying to get my attention, but all I wanted to do was obliterate it.

The healing ceremony took place in a tepee, around a large fire. The ceremony started at eight in the evening and lasted until sunrise. The group of about forty people chanted and prayed all night. During the ceremony we were given peyote, which was referred to as "medicine." The medicine man told me that this medicine would help heal me.

I had many of my friends sitting by me during the ceremony. Some had come from California and others from Colorado. Once I started journeying into my fear, their support helped me open myself up and stay with what I was experiencing. Without their support, I would never have been able to take this journey.

My senses became extremely heightened as I started delving into my fear. Every emotion that surfaced was experienced with extreme intimacy and clarity. After I had taken the peyote and participated in the invocation of the ceremony, the normal barriers that had stopped me from connecting to myself were instantly released.

As I chanted and stared endlessly into the fire, I began to feel a cold and dark force surrounding me. The sound of the drum and the rattles brought me into a trance where I could see this energy in the fire. The energy looked like a haunting dark mask outlined by red flames. Its eyes drew me in like a tornado. I actually felt a physical pulling on my body and I immediately tried to run away, but my friend who was sitting next to me stopped me. Once you enter the tepee, you are committed to staying there until the ceremony is over in the morning.

Once I sat back down, I took many deep breaths and looked into the fire again. This time I felt a sense of peace instead of fear. It was then that I was guided to close my eyes and connect with the many limited ideas I had about myself. I made contact with the tormented self-image that had guided most of my life. As I connected with this broken sense of self, a stream of traumatic images from my past began to be brought forth.

I made contact with every moment in my life whenI had been hurt and broken. I could see images of myself having surgery, receiving humiliating testosterone shots, and hearing the doctors tell me that I would always be infertile. Instead of denying the pain and embarrassment from these events like I usually had done, I began to give them love and acceptance. This was a very important moment in my healing journey. Once I tended to my pain and hurt with love and tenderness, a major shift happened—my entire heart opened.

Immediately after my heart opened, I could feel the immense presence of Spirit emerging from deep within me. I felt as if my whole body was tingling from the inside. I was overwhelmed with pure love. I felt as if my heart had expanded and encompassed the entire universe.

I realized in these mystical moments that Spirit had always lived inside me and always will. I realized this Spirit is what created me and everything else—that nothing is separate from this Spirit—and that Spirit only knows love.

I also realized that I did not need to limit myself anymore. By letting Spirit manifest itself into my life, I could live my life with a stronger energy. I could transform myself with gentleness, appreciation, and love. I could view myself as a perfect manifestation of Spirit—and nothing less.

Turning Mundane Experience into Sacred Experience

When you dedicate your life to the life of Spirit, all separateness dissolves. Your separateness is created by your inability to live in the present moment. If you approach your life in a way that separates yourself from the perfection of what is, you never experience the blessing of being whole.

When you experience a state of being whole, you experience perfect health. The words healthy and whole really mean the same thing, which is to be in a state of perfect rhythm and flow—a harmonious free flow of energy. This harmonious movement casts away any stagnancy that blocks your connection to life. The biggest and most detrimental stagnancy is created when you do not engage in the present moment. If you are not fully engaged in the present moment, you become lost in your thinking mind, which is always preoccupied with the past and future. Your thinking mind is always attached to what used to be or what could be. It is rarely satisfied with the simplicity of what is. This attachment creates a huge gap between yourself and Spirit and it literally halts the harmonious flow of energy inside of yourself.

Only when you open your heart to the perfection of the present moment can you nurture your connection to Spirit and experience a state of perfect wholeness. This connection is only possible when you harness the energy that flows from the center of your life. You do not need to look anywhere for Spirit—it is always within you and continually around you.

Inviting Spirit into your life is the fifth gateway toward healing. This is when you discover the key to living a spiritual life is in learning how to turn your mundane experience into sacred experience. As you learn to look for Spirit in everyday life, the veil that separates you from experiencing divinity will eventually disappear. Pema Chodron further illustrates this point: "There isn't anything except your own life that can be used as ground for your spiritual practice. Spiritual practice is your life, twenty-four hours a day."

If you are always searching for something, you will never find it—especially when what you are looking for is right inside you. Once you realize this very important truth, you will free yourself up to engage in your ordinary, everyday experience. It is here where you open yourself to the simple yet profound teachings of life.

Life is your greatest teacher. It is always providing you with invaluable lessons for personal growth. These lessons are to be found while washing the dishes, taking care of your children, listening to a friend tell a story, taking a walk, or enjoying a sunset. When you open your eyes to see the beauty in everyday life, you sanctify your connection to all things.

The way I was able to stay present and open myself to receive the lessons during the time that I was sick was by creating an inner sanctuary where nothing could disturb me. This sanctuary can be likened to your home inside—a home where you always feel safe, protected, and taken care of. There is a line in a song that I sing for the celebration of the Shabbat, which eloquently states, "When I call on the light of my soul, I come home." Every time I sing this line, I feel myself opening the door to my inner sanctuary.

Many times while driving myself to the hospital for chemotherapy treatments, I would start having anxiety attacks. Because of the intense trauma experienced during previous trips, my mind could hardly bear the thought of the upcoming visit. Stepping into the front door of the hospital was even more challenging. My body would start to shake and I would feel like I was about to throw up. The many distinct smells and sounds in the hospital made me want to run far, far away. The only way I could bring myself up to the tenth floor to receive my treatments was to connect with my inner sanctuary. I would imagine a great warm sun embracing and enveloping me. I would imagine this sun filling my entire body with radiance and peace. After doing this visualization, I would almost instantly feel that I could handle whatever came my way. I recently wrote a poem entitled "The Golden Castle," in which I describe how this inner sanctuary has nurtured and helped me.

When time is no longer time
And my mind is no longer a barrier
Then I will perceive your beauty
Unspoken yet overflowing
With words

When these dreams are no longer dreams
And my desires are nothing but inner strength
And conviction
Then I will caress your divinity
That crosses every border of longing
And enters into the limitless

When my pain is no longer pain
But an infinite opening into stillness
And the fierce winds of insecurity
Finally dissipate and are forgotten
Then I will enter into the golden castle
Of your devotion
And rest my head in your lap
Forgetting every part of my broken self

Once you learn to live every day from this inner sanctuary, you will able to be anywhere, in any moment, and sanctify it with your presence. This is how a great person such as Nelson Mandela was able to endure a long prison sentence and still maintain his dignity and presence. He could have been broken apart by his solitary confinement, his prison cell, the horrific treatment, but instead he transformed his prison cell into a sacred space where he was able to meditate and connect with the higher power of truth and love. In the uplifting book *Passionate Presence*, author Catherine Ingram states: "…and yet there is a sanctuary. It is not in the circumstances of the world but in the recognition of the silence that contains it. This silence is our own deep and true nature, and we can visit it or live in it any time we remember to do so."

Immaculée Ilibagiza's story is another amazing testimony to the existence of an inner sanctuary. As I mentioned in the last chapter, her book *Left to Tell* describes her personal experiences surviving the Rwandan holocaust. During this time, she was forced into hiding because of the unbelievable brutality all around her—over a million people were killed in only three months. The only way she could survive was to hide—and this is exactly what she did—for almost three months. She hid with seven other women in a tiny bathroom that probably should have fit, at the most, two to three people. Not only were these seven women unable to speak or whisper a word, but they were also unable to move, because killers would come by almost every day looking for them. Instead of feeling completely broken and torn apart, which I am sure would have been extremely easy to do, Immaculee Ilibagiza retreated into her inner sanctuary where she communed with the healing presence of God. In her own amazing words:

> I sat stone still on that dirty floor for hours on end, contemplating the purity of His energy while the force of His love flowed through me like a sacred river, cleansing my soul and easing my mind.... I surrendered my thoughts to God every day when I retreated to that special place in my heart to communicate with Him. That place was like a little slice of heaven, where my heart spoke to His holy spirit, and His spirit spoke to my heart.... In the midst of the genocide, I'd found my salvation. I knew that my bond with God would transcend the bathroom, the war, and the holocaust...

This inner sanctuary is the bridge that will connect you to the source of your being, and by connecting to the source of your being, you connect to the source of all creation. Just as all rivers flow into and come from the ocean, all beings flow into and come from the source.

Once you begin to drink from this ever-present wellspring of Spirit, you are able to confront any situation and turn it into a sacred experience. Again in the words of author Marcel Proust, "The voyage of discovery is not in seeking new landscapes but in having new eyes." Once you develop new eyes that are bathed in spiritual wisdom, you will be able to turn plain stones into radiant jewels and challenging moments into mystical experiences.

WHEN YOU ACCESS
The source
And follow
Its course
You flow
Like a river
Always at ease
You stand
Like a mountain
Always at peace
You welcome
Every experience
As it comes
Always giving
Yourself away
Like the sun
With its rays
Lighting
And embracing
And welcoming
Each new day

Prayer

Prayer is one of the strongest ways to transform your ordinary experience into spiritual experience. The best explanation I have found of how prayer helps to manifest health and wholeness is in Masaru Emoto's book, *The Hidden Messages in Water.*

This book eloquently describes how everything in the universe exists as vibration. It is through vibration that life expresses itself. He states, "The entire universe is in a state of vibration, and each thing generates its own frequency, which is unique...Human beings are also vibrating, and each individual vibrates at a unique frequency."

He goes on to state that all vibration creates a sound that emanates from within it. "The fact that everything is in a state of vibration also means that everything is creating sound." His enlightened discovery concerning vibration had to do with exposing water to different vibrational energies, which consisted of many different words or sounds, to see how these vibrations would influence the water. For example, he took the words "love" and "hate" and placed each word on its own container of water. He then took pictures of the water in an ice crystal form to see how these words affected the shape, form, and basic constitution of the water. He discovered that these vibrational energies directly impacted the water in astounding ways. The water that had the word "love" attached to it emitted a very beautiful, symmetric, and extremely ornate crystal that resembled an exquisite mandala, while the water that had the word "hate" attached to it emitted a very scattered, dissembled, and chaotic ice crystal.

He discovered that "as sound is created, there is a master listener to receive the sound: water ... water has the ability to copy and memorize information." Because water makes up most of your body, you can directly influence your health by sending healing vibrations into your body. The most healing vibration available to you is prayer. When prayer is spoken out loud, it can become even stronger. Masaru Emoto further describes this: "In Japan, it is said that words of the soul reside in a spirit called *kotodama*, or the spirit of words, and the act of speaking words has the power to change the world ... Words are an expression of the soul. And the condition of our soul is very likely to have an enormous impact on the water that composes as much as 70 percent of our body, and this impact will in no small way affect our bodies."

For thousands of years in India and in the East, they have used mantras to promote health and healing and a deep connection to Spirit. A mantra is simply a prayer that is stated out loud. These mantras are root sounds that vibrate at a very high frequency. When you say these mantras out loud, they instantly harmonize the energy of the body, mind, and spirit.

The reason this vibration is able to harmonize one's entire being is due to the existence of the human body's subtle energy system. In Hinduism, this subtle energy system is called the seven chakras. The seven chakras are centers of consciousness that directly influence the health of the entire body. These centers guide the health and well-being of your internal organs, as well as every system within the body. The chakras start at the base of the spine and go all the way up to the top of the head. Although I will not go into an extensive explanation of each chakra here, it is important to note that each chakra has a specific root sound that balances it. When chanted out loud, these root sounds harmonize the chakras instantly and bring a state of peace and well-being to the physical body. You may ask, "How is this really possible? How can saying some words out loud heal my body?" Well, as I mentioned previously through Masaru Emoto's wonderful example, everything in the universe is made up of specific vibrations, and because each vibration has a unique frequency, you can learn to influence and balance each of them through the use of the healing harmonies of sound. Since sound is pure vibration, it has the potential to directly harmonize every frequency it comes in contact with.

During the time that I was sick, I spent a lot of my time in the hospital playing a dulcimer and chanting. It was the only thing that really relaxed me. The funny thing was, it would also relax anyone else who could hear it. Other patients and nurses would sometimes come sit in my room just to be near the chanting. Everyone, no matter what their belief system or what they may have thought about the specific prayers I was chanting, could feel this healing vibration.

There are many different ways of chanting. You don't necessarily need to learn how to chant; you can simply choose different words or prayers, and then say them out loud. Sometimes I just repeat the words "love" and "peace," which are very powerful mantras in their own right.

You can also create your own prayers. While I was going through one of my hardest days of chemotherapy, a nurse in the hospital told me the Serenity Prayer, which reads: "God grant me the serenity to accept the things I cannot change, the courage to change the things I can, and the wisdom to know the difference."

The next morning as I started reciting the Serenity Prayer, I began to think of my own version of it, which I now use every day as part of my morning prayers:

> *God, grant me the serenity*
> *To be peaceful*
> *To move gracefully*
> *On this Earth*
> *To generate a sense of worth*
> *For myself and for all of life*
> *And thereby removing*
> *Unnecessary strife*
>
> *Grant me the courage*
> *To live my truth each day*
> *To follow my bliss*

To embrace my experience
In whichever way
It takes me
And thereby opening myself
Continually without delay

Grant me the wisdom
To endure life's uncertainty
To open my heart to possibility
To strengthen my capacity
To be aware
And thereby always living

In a state of prayer

Creating your own prayers is another effective way of transforming your mundane experience into sacred experience. A prayer that you write and then say out loud has the power to help free you from whatever everyday struggles you may be experiencing. For example, perhaps you are struggling with having compassion for a friend who recently hurt you and who is now going through a hard time. Maybe, at this time, you do not feel capable of calling him up on the phone or going out with him. Instead you can write and say a prayer for him. The prayer could sound something like this: "May (your friend's name) be protected and guided by divine love during this challenging time. May (he or she) experience peace during this time. May it be so." The feeling that the prayer generates will help you to refocus your attention in an uplifting and positive manner, which in turn will help create a space for healing your relationship with your friend, as well as helping to draw support into your friend's situation.

The use of prayer helps refocus your body and mind's energy. It takes our incessant need to gravitate to the negative (fear) and replaces it with the healing force of the positive (love). When you speak loving and compassionate words, you instantly draw the power of Spirit into your space and the space of whomever you are sending this energy to. These loving and compassionate words, spoken with a pure intention, will charge your being on so many levels.

Perhaps the biggest reason prayer and the use of healing sound is so effective is because it harnesses the power of your emotion. Whereas at the third gateway you learned to work through and release emotion, in the later gateways you learn how to harness spiritually charged emotions to consistently connect to the power of Spirit.

Your emotion is the tool that allows you to resonate with the highest vibration possible—the vibration of love. The presence of love is the presence of Spirit— they are one and the same. By embracing the emotion of love, you awaken the strongest spiritual presence available to you. This spiritual presence opens you to receive your life in a completely new way. This way is the way of the mystic. Mystics allow the presence of the divine to inspire and energize their entire being with spiritual awareness. This spiritual awareness is what allows you to experience the mystery of life with endless wonder and awe. This spiritual awareness is the fuel that turns every day and every moment into a cause for great prayer and celebration.

How to Enter this Gateway:
Nurture Your Spirit

When you awaken the powerful energy of Spirit in your life, you learn how to transcend every limitation imaginable. This is because Spirit does not know limitations. As I stated previously, Spirit has infinite potential and is endlessly creative. And because Spirit is what you are, you too have infinite potential and are endlessly creative.

Awakening this presence is only possible when you learn how to nurture your connection to your higher self. As I have described previously, the bridge that connects you to this healing space is your inner sanctuary. Your inner sanctuary can be likened to your home inside—the place where you feel completely at peace.

The way that this inner sanctuary is best accessed is through a sacred space where you invoke healing energy. This sacred space helps nurture you in every way imaginable. It removes any extraneous activities—such as answering the telephone or thinking about worldly concerns—and helps you to home in and focus on the energy of your spirit.

SACRED SPACE
Is the place
Where you forget
All the busyness
Laying to rest
Any thoughts of dis-ease
Or illness
Creating eternal time
By drawing a circle
Instead of lines
And lighting candles
That enlighten your mind
Awakening the Divine inside
And calling forth
Your legion of angels
That will ignite
Your own blissful light
And give you holy eyes
So that you may see
With God's healing sight

A sacred space helps you to tune into your higher self rather than your thinking self. When you spend your time focused on your higher self, you let go of anything that holds you back from focusing all your energy on the perfection of the present moment. This sacred space helps you attune yourself to this perfection by helping you calm and relax your thinking mind. Because your thinking mind likes to spend its time analyzing your experience, it never fully lets go to receive the divinity that is available in every new moment. Your thinking mind is always planning for the next thing, always suggesting that what you need is somehow out of reach. Once you are able to let go of this faulty thinking and instead tune into the sanctuary of your spirit, you will be able to fully let go into the present moment and experience a sense of great ease.

The famous mythologist Joseph Campbell called this sacred space your "bliss station." In order to energize and charge your spiritual battery, you need a spiritual station were you can do this. Joseph Campbell describes this bliss station as "a place where you can simply experience and bring forth what you are, and what you might be … at first you may find nothing is happening … but if you have a sacred place and use it, take advantage of it, something will happen."

A good way to create your sacred space is with a personal altar. An altar is a place where you can retreat from the chaos of the world and turn inwards and relax. It is a place where you can reconnect to your higher self.

By creating a beautiful space that is adorned with flowers and incense, it will immediately draw you inward to connect to your inner sanctuary. After you create your altar, you will want to start dedicating a certain amount of time each day to using it. The more time you spend there, the more spiritually energized you will feel.

Performing healing rituals is a great way to spend time at your altar. Healing rituals, like the one I experienced at the Native American ceremony, are powerful ways to connect with Spirit. Healing rituals have been done for thousands of years for a reason—they work! Native American teacher and shaman Sun Bear further describes how healing rituals miraculously work: "When humans participate in ceremony, they enter a sacred space. Everything outside of that space shrivels in importance. Time takes on a different dimension. Emotions flow more freely. The bodies of participants become filled with the energy of life, and this energy reaches out and blesses the creation around them. All is made new; everything becomes sacred."

A healing ritual consists of three distinct parts that complete and define it. The first part is the stating of your prayer and intention. A way that you can state your prayer is to light a candle. After you light the candle, you can say out loud what you intend to create in this healing space. By stating this prayer out loud, it helps to draw this vibrational energy into your space.

The second part is done when you bring forth your prayer through a conscious surrendering to the power of your emotions. As I have previously mentioned, your emotions hold a tremendous amount of power. They are your mystical keys to unlock all the closed doors and blocked passageways in your life. Your emotions are the power that confirms and upholds the integrity and conviction of your heart. It is only through your emotional state that you change your physical reality. In the words of Israel Regardie, author of *The Art of True Healing*, "Prayer is indispensable. The wish, the heart's desire, the goal to be reached, must be held firmly in mind, vitalized by divine power, and propelled forward into the universe by the fiery intensity of all the emotional exaltation we are capable of." At the second part of a healing ceremony, you must become the feeling inside your heart that surrounds your prayer. To think and ponder about your prayer is not enough—you must fully embody what your prayer feels like. If your prayer is to be healed, you must feel that you are already healed—you must live from the answer of what you intend to create—and then the presence of Spirit will come to your aid and help you to turn your prayer into a miracle.

The last part of the healing ritual is done through giving thanks to Spirit with a deep feeling of reverence and humility so that "thy will, will be done." This deep feeling of respect allows you to receive the miracle of your prayer without any judgments or expectations. In a newly translated version of the New Testament of the Bible, it states, "All things that you ask straightly, directly... From inside My name—You will be given... So ask without hidden motive and be surrounded by your answer—Be enveloped by what you desire, that your gladness be full."

Once you have completely embraced this feeling of humility and opened your heart to the presence and power of Spirit, allowing yourself to be "surrounded by your answer," you can then blow out your candle, which creates a sense of closure and completes the healing ritual.

Exercise: Healing Rituals

The power of ritual allows you to reunite all the separate and isolated parts of yourself. All inner imbalances stem from a feeling of separateness. This separateness tries to fool you with the illusion that you are not connected to Spirit. It tries to make you think that you are completely alone and thus have to fend for yourself. This "fending for yourself" is the root of all fear. The only way to release this fear is to reconnect to the unity of your whole and complete being, which means you connect to the healing presence of Spirit.

This next exercise should be done in front of a personal altar that you have created for yourself. An altar is easily set up with a little table that you put in a corner of your living room or bedroom. You can put a colorful cloth over the table and then put a candle and incense and flowers on the table. You can also include crystals and stones, photographs of spiritual teachers or family members, and anything else that makes you feel connected to Spirit.

This exercise follows the same structure for a healing ritual as I previously illustrated. Your healing ritual should be done in a quiet space where you will not be disturbed. You will need a candle and a bundle of some healing herbs that you can burn, such as sage or cedar.

First, I would like for you to sit down on the floor, or in a chair if that is more comfortable, and then close your eyes and internally state a prayer and intention that you would like to manifest. This prayer may be for healing a relationship, for healing a dis-ease, for closure to something that happened in your past, for forgiveness to someone that hurt you, or for strength and courage to persevere through a challenging time in your life. Whatever your prayer's purpose, it is important that you get a clear image in your mind of what you would like to manifest. For example, if you internally state: "I pray for healing my relationship with my father," you should then clearly see what that image of a healed relationship between you and your father looks like. With this image in your mind, you can then light the candle at your altar. After you light the candle, you then, with hands in prayer position, say your prayer out loud. This time, though, instead of stating "I pray for …" say, "My relationship to my father is healed." You can say this as many times as you feel necessary. Normally I say it three times.

The second part of the healing ritual takes place when you embody the feeling of what, in this case, would be a feeling of a renewed and healthy relationship to your father. As you sit in front of your altar, you nurture this feeling inside of yourself by continuing to visualize your father and you in a healed way. You sit for however long is necessary for this feeling to arise. As I previously mentioned, it is the power of your feeling that does the magic. Your feeling is what opens you to Spirit and allows Spirit to then manifest this miracle into your life.

Finally, after you are able to sustain this feeling for at least five to ten minutes, light your bundle of purifying herbs and then wave it around your body while saying, "May it be so." You can say this as many times as you like. After you do this, you can then say a statement of respect that reflects your gratitude to Spirit for allowing this miracle to unfold. I like to say, "I am thankful for Spirit for allowing my life to unfold with grace. I am thankful for Spirit for awakening me to my divine self. I am thankful for Spirit for guiding me in all ways." After you thank the presence of Spirit, you can then blow out the candle, which completes your healing ritual.

The Message of this Gateway: Cultivate Sacred Space

Sacred space is the place where you willfully draw Spirit into you. It is the force of Spirit that allows you to live your life in a holy way. When you harness this energy, you turn every moment of your life into a blessing.

Once you awaken to the realization that nothing is separate from Spirit, you will learn to see divinity within all of creation—even in the most challenging of circumstances. You are capable of transforming any place into a sacred space. Your great power lies in connecting with Spirit and allowing its overflowing abundance to nourish your entire life.

JOY

LET GO OF FEAR AND YOU
instantaneously realize love.
Let go of hurt and you
instantaneously realize peace.
Let go of yourself and you
instantaneously realize bliss.

Once the presence of Spirit has awakened within you, the next two gateways literally swing right open as if a great healing wind has blown into your life. As Spirit awakens deep within, you unfold the two most spiritual experiences—the experience of love and the experience of peace. At the sixth gateway, you experience a great love that nourishes and sustains your entire being, while at the seventh gateway you experience a great peace that blesses your life with an inner realization of who you truly are.

At the sixth gateway, where you open yourself to the experience of love, your life begins to overflow with an abundance of joy. Again in the wise and eloquent words of Don Miguel Ruiz: "When you have the courage to open your heart completely to love, a miracle happens. You start perceiving the reflection of your love in everything. Then eating, walking, talking, singing, dancing, showering, working, playing—everything you do becomes a ritual of love. When everything becomes a ritual of love, you are no longer thinking; you are feeling and enjoying your life. You find pleasure in every activity you do because you love to do it. Just to be alive is wonderful, and you feel intensely happy."

This happiness and joy is the direct result of having fully let go of yourself. The presence of love allows you to let go of the tight grip you have on yourself, because at this stage in your spiritual journey, you realize that there is nothing more to hold on to. The presence of fear is what had previously forced you into thinking that you needed to desperately hold on to and control life, but this was only because you hadn't experienced this all-pervasive love from deep within your being. This awakening of divine love now allows you to feel safe and protected enough to let every part of yourself go. While at the second gateway you learned how to refine your responses to life by letting go of control of a situation, at the sixth gateway you learn how to let go of complete control of yourself, which means letting go of your ego. This letting go of the ego is what lets in an experience of divine love. This feeling of complete surrender releases the controlling grip that your ego has had on you and allows you to simply enjoy your life. I love Rachel Naomi Remen's words that further illustrate this: "Blessing life may be more about learning how to celebrate life than learning how to fix life. It may require an appreciation of life as it is and an acceptance of much in life that we cannot understand. It may mean developing an eye for joy."

When you have "developed an eye for joy," you allow things to fall into place, as they will, because no matter what your experiences are, you joyfully experience all of them. Through your growing feeling of joy, you begin to feel extremely blessed for everything that comes your way. Thus, everything in your life takes on new meaning—everything becomes an opportunity to experience more and more joy—even in the face of difficulty.

As I described in the Trust chapter, two weeks before my daughter was born, I was told that I had a recurrence of testicular cancer in my lymph nodes. I was told that I would need to undergo three months of intense chemotherapy, during which I would need to stop working.

I was completely distraught and upset about how the chemotherapy would affect me and my ability to take care of my family. For the two weeks before my daughter was born, I was a wreck. I was living in a whirlwind of stress. Caught up in calls to social services, family members, and friends, I had forgotten about the joy of being with my wife and anticipating the birth of our child.

It wasn't until the day of her birth that I began to let go and let in the magic and joy of her arrival. Because my daughter's birth was a home birth and I had a major role, I had to be completely present. I had to push on my wife's back to help support her, as well as cut the umbilical cord and catch my baby as she was being born.

During the entire birthing process, I had completely forgotten about cancer. I had also forgotten about money and work. My mind was on one thing—my daughter.

As my daughter was being born, my entire body felt rushes of joy. I felt so overwhelmed by the experience that I started to cry. I had never felt such joy before. I cried and cried. My tears were tears of joy and gratitude.

After the birth, I went to the grocery store to get her first package of diapers and as I was walking in the aisles I remember thinking to myself that I was the luckiest man in the world. Even though I had just been told that I had a recurrence of cancer, I knew in my heart that all that mattered was how I was feeling right at that moment—which was ecstatic. I knew that nothing in the world could take this feeling away from me.

This overwhelming feeling of joy helped me forget every last bit of my despair. I no longer cared to worry or become anxious about my family's situation because I was too busy enjoying my life. Around this time, I had been reading a great book by Joseph Campbell, which stated, "Find a place inside where there's joy, and the joy will burn out the pain." Those words were such an inspiration that I posted them up on my wall. Every day, they helped me stay focused on what truly mattered.

In the challenging weeks ahead, my daughter, Malana Elizabeth, continually helped me stay present and joyful. The more I let go and experienced the pure miracle of her presence, the more I was able to gracefully endure my chemotherapy treatments.

As I continued to let go into my situation and experience more and more joy, I began to realize how absolutely blessed I was. Through this feeling of being blessed

I continued to become even more blessed. In the following weeks after my daughter's birth, I received a phone call from the director of the preschool where I had previously worked. She enthusiastically told me that the preschool had raised more than $3,000 for my family and me. After I got off the phone, I looked at my wife and I began to laugh and cry at the same time. Even in the face of such a difficult and trying situation, life was still overflowing with joy and abundance.

Laughter

Kahlil Gibran, the famous Lebanese poet, once said, "I would not exchange the laughter of my heart for the fortunes of the multitudes; nor would I be content with converting my tears, invited by my agonized self, into calm. It is my fervent hope that my whole life on this earth will ever be in tears and laughter." When you let yourself go into the experience of life, the experience overwhelms you with "tears and laughter" that flow from an ever-growing feeling of joy in your soul. This joy continually reminds you how blessed you truly are.

My father was able to achieve this experience of joy in one of the most challenging of life's circumstances. As I mentioned before, my father recently passed away from ALS. I watched this disease take away every part of his physical freedoms, completely paralyzing him within three years of the diagnosis. While this was happening,

A SMILE IS ALL
That it takes
To learn
From your mistakes
Give thanks
And embrace
The possibility
Of change
And the willingness
To turn the page
And take what is old
And make it new
To look into the past
With a different
Point of view
And to make friends
With what continually
Challenges you

he also knew that the eventual outcome of this horrible disease would be death.

During this incredibly difficult time, my father maintained his sense of dignity. This dignity was brilliantly achieved because he was able to fully let go of himself. He was able to surrender himself and his situation to a power greater than himself. He was able to take the focus off of his need for security and comfort and let go into the mystery of life.

This sense of ease that he was able to cultivate with the disease and with life lightened his load considerably. My father's heart was filled to the brim with laughter and joy. He would joke about almost everything. He would also tell stories about his youth and would continually express his gratitude for life.

My father had a lot of great phrases that he would say. One of my favorites was simply, "No tensing up." He would say this whenever he noticed that someone was holding on too tightly, creating unnecessary strain and difficulty for themselves. I believe the reason most people "tense up" is because they are unable to let go of themselves. Often we burden ourselves by thinking too much about work, money, cleaning the house, or even the somewhat contrived pressures on the "to do" lists. It is only when we let go of this unnecessary tension that we allow ourselves the freedom to laugh, to let go, and to experience great joy.

In Norman Cousins's book *The Anatomy of an Illness*, he describes how he healed himself of a life-threatening disease, ankylosing spondylitis, through a healthy dose of laughter. Part of his daily medicine consisted of watching Marx Brothers films and *Candid Camera*. It was through his joy and laughter that he achieved a state of perfect health. In his own words, "I made the joyous discovery that ten minutes of genuine belly laughter had an anesthetic effect and would give me at least two hours of pain-free sleep...When the pain-killing effect of the laughter wore off, we would switch on the motion picture projector again and not infrequently, it would lead to another pain-free interval."

Laughter is the pure expression of joy. It is the result of having completely let yourself go. When you laugh, you relax—and when you relax, you let go. In this way, there may be nothing more healing and conducive to your health than allowing yourself to laugh and smile. These expressions instantly give your body the message that you are healthy. In the book *Spiritual Aspects of the Healing Arts*, internationally acclaimed doctor and incredibly inspiring author and lecturer Bernie Siegel states, "The changes which create the environment conducive to healing are the introduction of laughter, music, and love.... then every cell in the body is involved in the healing process. When we laugh, every cell laughs. When we love, our immune system feels the most vibrant message it can receive and fights for our life."

The effect of laughter has been studied by scientists and revealed to have many physiological health benefits. One prominent health benefit is laughter's ability to lower the level of cortisol, a stress hormone, in the human body. Since stress drastically lowers the functioning of the immune system, making it one of the leading causes of disease, laughter may be one of the most powerful defenses we have.

Laughter also supplies the lungs with oxygen, stimulates the brain and the heart, and increases the natural killer cells that help to defend the immune system against cancer and other diseases.

The best way to stimulate laughter is to engage in play. Play is not just for kids. When you play, you let go of all your worry that stops you from enjoying the bliss and joy of the present moment. In the words of Jesus, "Unless you change and become like little children, you will never enter the kingdom of heaven." The "kingdom of heaven" *is* the bliss of the present moment.

One of the most healing things I do on a daily basis is dance with my three-year-old daughter. We put our favorite music on the stereo and dance and laugh and sing. It is my favorite part of the day. While dancing, I do not think about what I have to do or what I haven't done—I simply laugh and smile, and most importantly, I let go of myself. After about an hour of having let go of myself, I feel completely energized and renewed, knowing that my "love for living" battery was just completely charged.

Most people do not realize how powerful our play and laughter truly is. Playing and laughing rejuvenates your entire being. It helps you to not take yourself so seriously and, as my father would say, it helps you to "not tense up." Dr. O. Carl Simonton, internationally acclaimed oncologist, author, and speaker states, "When you're depressed, the whole body is depressed, and it translates to the cellular level. The first objective is to get your energy up, and you can do it through play. It's one of the most powerful ways of breaking up hopelessness and bringing energy into the situation."

It is imperative that you play and connect to joy each and every day of your life. When you are joyful, you do not become disillusioned by the many overwhelming challenges that life presents. By continuing to enjoy yourself in the face of adversity, you continue to affirm life's beauty.

When you smile, you don't focus on your mistakes or shortcomings. When you smile, you instantly embrace your life, with all of its hardship and difficulty. In Thich Nhat Hanh's words, "Smiling means that we are ourselves, that we are not drowned in forgetfulness. How can I smile when I am filled with so much sorrow? It is natural—you need to smile to your sorrow because you are more than your sorrow."

Humility

Humility is another way to embrace the joy in your life. You become humble when you are able to see beyond yourself and into a larger perspective of life. This requires that you stop your ego from controlling the way you experience life.

Make no mistake, the ego is necessary to function in the world. It helps you to pay your bills and shop at the grocery store, but if it tries to overpower your connection to life, you will forget who and what you really are.

An unhealthy ego responds to life by thinking that it is in control. It tries to dominate your mind and body with endless demands that will eventually rob you of your life-force energy. These demands take the form of all the "needs" that we think we must have to be happy. These "needs" are nothing but barriers that stand in the way of your blissful connection to Spirit. Power, control, and dominance are just a few of the outfits in the extensive wardrobe of the ego. The ego is delighted when you succumb to these emotions and uselessly strive to please it—but the ego is never pleased—it always wants more. Just look around and you can see that the entire world is an ego-driven mess. The reason the world is so toxic is because most people serve their egos instead of Spirit. With the ego, everything becomes chaotic and destructive. With Spirit, everything becomes whole and peaceful.

Only when you surrender your ego through a feeling of humility can you develop your spiritual presence. Humility instantly rids you of the toxic and draining presence of the ego—the presence that tries to make you believe that you have to search for happiness outside of yourself. The presence of humility is what allows you to let go of this inauthentic way of living your life.

HUMILITY IS BOWING DOWN

To the simplicity of now
And realizing that
You are not bound
By false connections
That try to throw you further
Into separation
Tying you into the ego's
Heavy chains
That will try
To wrap around you
Creating more pain
By making you hide
In sorrow and fear
But you know
That you have a great light
Stored deep inside
Just waiting for you
To arrive
To grab hold and unfold
Its magnificent road
That will eventually lead you
Away from fearful control
And into the healing presence
Of your soul

Due to the many physical traumas that I have experienced, I have often struggled with my ego. On many occasions, it has tried to make me feel how imperfect my body is and how I must fix it in order to feel better about myself. It has tried to tell me that I always need something else to fix my broken self. It has continually tried to fool me with the idea that something is always wrong with me. After wrestling with this internal judge (the ego) for a long time, I finally realized the only thing wrong with me was that my ego was out of control and trying to rule my life. Again in the wise words of Deepak Chopra: "If you want to reach a state of bliss, then go beyond your ego ... Make a decision to relinquish the need to control, the need to be approved, and the need to judge. Those are the three things the ego is doing all the time. It's very important to be aware of them every time they come up."

Once you humbly let go of yourself—which means letting go of the need to be approved, the need to judge, and the need to have more and more needs—you are delivered into an uplifted state of grace. Grace is the power in your life that allows you to feel that you are being carried and supported by an unseen force. You only experience this force when you let in the abundant energy of Spirit. When you let go of the limited energy of your ego and instead allow the infinite power of Spirit to move through you, you witness the unfolding of this grace—and through this unfolding you are led into a

WHEN YOU FOCUS
On giving
Instead of getting
Then you forget
To put your expectations
Onto things
And you forget
To worry about
Always being
In control
'Cause you
Continuously practice
The sacred art
Of letting go
Where you spend
All of your time
Opening your heart
And opening your soul
And making room
For miracles
To grow

connection to life more powerful than anything you will ever encounter.

When you connect with the "healing presence of your soul," you relinquish your need to forcefully conquer the present moment. When you experience the abundant energy of Spirit—the abundant energy of your soul—you enter the present moment without any baggage. This baggage can take the form of many unhealthy attachments—the knee-jerk, ego-driven reactions such as jealousy, pride, greed, criticism, and lust—that try to limit your experience of love and make you feel that you do not deserve to feel good about yourself. If you get caught up in these false notions of the ego, you act as though something is inherently wrong with you and thus forget how to laugh and smile and let yourself go.

Fully letting yourself go is the only way you experience true joy. The ego is defenseless in the presence of pure love and joy because love and joy instantly remove every burdensome illusion created by the ego. Don't be fooled—these illusions are, to quote one of my poems, the "heavy chains that try to wrap around you, creating more pain." You throw off and remove these "chains" (the ego-driven attachments listed above) when you release your ego's needs for security and comfort and instead focus on being nourished by the abundant and unlimited energy of Spirit. This presence of Spirit instantly connects you to joy, because you inwardly feel how much divinity lives within you. This feeling makes you want to completely give of yourself, because you already feel that you have so much. It is this attitude of giving that expresses your humility and your gratitude for life. Again in Kahlil Gibran's words, "There are those who have little and give it all. These are the believers in life and the bounty of life, and their coffer is never empty." When you fully give, you receive and receive and receive. You receive miracles. The miracle of now. The miracle of love. The miracle of life.

When you fully give of yourself, you have no expectations of what should or shouldn't be; you simply see things as they are. Seeing things as they are allows you to be fully present and removes the false eyes that the ego tries to deceive you with. Once you remove the blinders of your ego, you are able to completely let yourself go. This miraculous act of letting yourself go gives birth to an enlightened and wakeful presence that is always grateful, always humble, always open to experiencing the great joy that continually surrounds you.

How to Enter this Gateway: Experience Love

Once you have become open and vulnerable to joy, you experience the power of grace that opens your heart to receive divine love. This divine love flows from the source of your being. It is pure, untainted, and unconditional.

If you were to view the spiritual journey in the image of a flower, the seed would represent Spirit, the stem and the leaves would represent the power of life, and the flower petals and their beauty would represent the blossoming of divine love. Once you realize your source (the seed) and allow the power of life to nurture and help you grow (the stem and leaves), you experience the unfolding of your inherent divinity—which opens up divine love (the flower petals).

In order to experience this divine unfolding, you need to pass through the same three steps as the metaphor of the flower. First, you need to work through your fear and connect to the source of your being. Second, you need to humbly let go of your ego and open yourself to the power of life. And lastly, you need to open your heart to receive the grace and splendor of divine love.

Once you feel this blossoming of love inside, you will know that you have connected to the source and have allowed the power of life to gracefully move through you. When you live life from this sacred place, you continually bless everyone and everything around you. If you have ever gone to see a saint or a spiritual master, you would notice that they spend most of their time blessing people. Because of their deep connection to Spirit and their unlimited reservoir of divine love, their desire to bless people flows naturally from within them.

This divine love has the power to heal any dis-ease. It has the power to cut through any imbalance or internal block and restore harmony and peace within everything that it touches. Internationally acclaimed author and revolutionary physician Larry Dossey, author of *Healing Words* and *Prayer is Good Medicine*, further illustrates the power of love to heal your life: "The power of love to change bodies is legendary, built into folklore, common sense, and everyday experience. Love moves the flesh, it pushes matter around."

When you access divine love, you fill your life with miracles. You are able to make the impossible, possible. You are able to make the unbelievable, believable. You are able to make the unhealthy, healthy.

My daughter was a miracle that blessed me because of the love that I had generated inside myself. I had spent half my life disbelieving that I could ever have a child. Since I was told at the age of fourteen that I would remain infertile for the rest of my life, I was always cutting myself down with unloving thoughts. When I met my wife, I was still very much consumed by these negative thoughts. My wife, who is the sweetest woman I've ever met, spent almost all of our time together complimenting me. She would always tell me how beautiful I was and how she believed in me and how she knew that I would one day give her a baby. For many months, I shrugged off her compliments and vehemently insisted that I could never have a child and that I would never amount to anything in my life. But my wife persisted in showering me with love—and one day it finally got through. I can remember the day very well. I woke up early in the morning, watching the sun come up through our window in our studio apartment. I was staring at a tree that stood outside the window and admiring how the light touched the branches. Above the window was a hanging crystal that illuminated a little rainbow onto my chest. I was instantly enamored. I felt a warmth and a joy inside of myself that I hadn't experienced since I was a child. I looked over at my wife, who was sleeping next to me, and silently thanked her. I knew that it was her unconditional love for me that helped me to finally wake up and embrace the love within myself. I got out of the bed and smiled with such gratitude. I walked around our little apartment as if it were the first time. I touched our plants, I continued to stare out the window, I smiled at our photographs, and I lit a candle at our altar with the intention that I would always hold this love within me. When my wife woke up, I immediately told her that I would one day give her a child. Inwardly, I knew that this feeling of love inside of me was capable of any miracle, and within three and a half weeks this miracle came true—my wife had become pregnant!

Emmett Fox, author of *Power Through Constructive Thinking*, further describes love's miraculous healing power:

> There is no difficulty that enough love will not conquer. No disease that enough love will not heal. No door that enough love will not open. No gulf that enough love will not bridge. No wall that enough love will not throw down. No sin that enough love will not redeem.
>
> It makes no difference how deeply seated may be the trouble. How hopeless the outlook. How muddled the tangle. How great the mistake. A sufficient realization of love will dissolve it all. If only one could love enough, you would be the happiest and most powerful being in the world.

At the sixth gateway, the power of love moves through you with lightning speed as you learn to continually re-generate yourself through the joyful practice of giving and receiving love. In the words of the great fourteenth-century Persian poet Hafiz, "We are people who need to love, because love is the soul's life. Love is simply cre-ation's greatest joy." This practice of giving and receiv-ing love not only makes being alive fun and exciting, but it is what gives your life true meaning and purpose. In the musician James Taylor's inspiring words, "The secret of life is enjoying the passage of time." When you spend your time "enjoying the passage of time," you are always engaged with the experience of love. Whether you are at work or with your family or spending time in nature by yourself, you completely give of every part of yourself through your experience of this joy and love, because your experience of joy naturally and inevitably touches everyone and everything around you. Your joy and love are actually contagious. They provide a great warmth to all those that you share your life with. I cannot think of a better gift to give someone than this extremely inspired and uplifted presence. You will find that the more you develop and give this presence to others, the more you will also receive. This humble and joyful presence opens you to receive an intimacy with life that will fill your life with overflowing abundance. As your love grows and matures through this intimacy, it will turn into a great power that will heal you. Through experiencing such bliss, you will sanctify every day of your life with your own inner light. When you share this inner light with others, you create a radiance so bright that it has the power to heal the entire world.

Exercise: Working with Prayer

Love mends all. Only love can make whatever is broken whole again. With love as your deepest prayer, you allow miracles to unfold. There is a great passage from the book *A Course in Miracles* that states, "Prayer is the medium of miracles ... Through prayer love is received, and through miracles love is expressed." This quote is a great passageway into the next exercise, which focuses on using prayer as the medium to give and receive love.

As I have previously mentioned, prayer is the medium by which you reconnect yourself to Spirit. Prayer is the humble bridge that you construct that allows the immense presence of Spirit to enter into your heart. The way that I like to pray is with my hands together, palms facing each other, placed directly in front of my heart, and with a smile on my face. Both the placement of your hands and your smile are indicators to Spirit that you are open, ready, and willing to be a participant in the holy act of giving and receiving love.

I would like for you to pick a quiet time of the day and a quiet place where you can practice this next exercise. Sit down on the floor with a cushion or sit comfortably in a chair. I would like for you to think of one person, one external event, and one internal issue that you struggle with. After you have gotten a clear idea of these three challenges, you can then place your hands together in prayer position and, with a smile on your face, begin with the first healing prayer for the person you chose and state, "I smile to (the person you chose)." After you state this, I would like for you to visualize this person receiving your smile and then this person smiling back at you. I would like you to hold this feeling and visualization for at least five minutes. Then I would like you to proceed to the next healing prayer for the external event. I would like you to state, "I smile to (the external event that you chose)." I would like you to visualize yourself in the external event with a smile on your face and an ease in your heart. I would like for you to hold this feeling and visualization for at least five minutes. Lastly, I would like for you to send a healing prayer to yourself. Please state, "I smile to (the internal issue you chose)." I would like for you to visualize yourself completely letting go of this issue and continuing to smile as you do so. See yourself free from all struggle and full of only love and peace. Again, hold this visualization for at least five minutes.

After you have done the above visualizations, I would like for you to close this exercise by stating this affirmation three times: "I let go of my ego that tries to limit my experience of love and I let in boundless, pure, unconditional love. I choose to focus all of my energy on this great healing love."

The Message of this Gateway:
Let Go and Let In

You create an abundance of joy when you let go of every part of yourself. When you let yourself completely go, you awaken your heart to the experience of perfect, unconditional love. By connecting to this great love, you transcend every part of your ego and your fear-based responses that hold you back from experiencing true health and wholeness.

Perhaps the greatest work you can do in your life is to allow this energy of love and joy to flow through you. This healing energy will open your heart to receive endless blessings from Spirit. These blessings sustain your life with a continual reminder of how precious your life is. When you live your life from this humble and open place, you turn every day into a magical and wondrous celebration.

Contentment

FOLLOW YOUR BREATH
and journey into now.
Follow your heart
and journey into love.
Follow your soul
and journey into peace.

At the seventh gateway, after grounding yourself in acceptance and trust, working through and then transforming your suffering, unfolding your highest truth and the power of compassion, connecting to the presence of Spirit, and experiencing the great love and joy that flows from deep within your being, you are delivered into the land of your soul. Your soul is your essence. It is the place deep inside where you feel perfectly and honestly yourself.

Throughout your life, it can become very easy to lose touch with your essence. This essence can be defined as your core, and often this core gets covered over and forgotten about. A good metaphor for this is the image of an onion, with the core of the onion being your soul, and all the layers around it being the many false identifications that hide your true nature. Once you remove these thick layers of doubt, fear, and insecurity that you have unwillingly placed onto yourself, you rediscover the essence of who and what you are.

In your soul-space, there is never any doubt about who you are. Oftentimes, little children live from their soul-space, which is why they are always incredibly present and open. They are also extremely intuitive, sensitive, and perceptive. These are all qualities that stem from living from your soul-space. When you connect with your soul-space, you always live life in the here-and-now and this instantly brings you to a place of profound inner knowing.

Your soul is your own unique expression of Spirit that is eternal, interconnected to all things, perfect, and whole. When you connect to this presence, you unfold a wisdom that transcends the physical limitations of this world. You are able to feel and see things beyond your normal senses. You are also able to heal and renew yourself in every way imaginable. This profound state of inner knowing becomes stronger and stronger the more you allow your soul to be in contact with your mind—continually informing and reminding it of who and what you really are—which is an eternal, interconnected, perfect, and whole being.

The only real dis-ease and imbalance is when you lose touch with your soul and instead identify yourself as anything but God or Spirit. Your physical existence suffers greatly when you focus all your energy on the external world rather than your internal world. If you disconnect yourself from your internal world through a false identification with the external, you will live in exile from the land of your soul, and be forever lost. It is only through continual contact with your soul (internal world) that the external world takes on any meaning.

The external world is the realm of the material world—your body, the earth, and all the things of this world—and this world cannot exist without the internal world, the realm of the soul and of God, continually informing, guiding, and supporting it. Your understanding of this relationship is crucial in terms of fulfilling your healing journey. Once you understand that the internal form always dictates the external shape of things, you realize that you can heal any illness, mend any relationship, and bring harmony and peace to any situation. This is because, as it is stated in the Bible in the Gospel of Matthew, "With God, all things are possible."

You can empower your internal world to harmoniously influence your external world. At the seventh gateway, this harmonious relationship unfolds as you learn to cultivate this space of being rather than a space of doing. Doing so will nourish your life. When you engage with doing, you spend your time always trying to shield yourself from life—always trying to occupy yourself, so you don't have to turn inward and self-reflect. When you engage with a space of being, though, you allow yourself the freedom to look inward to find true peace and contentment.

Once you awaken this healing presence by looking within yourself and cultivating a space of being, you stop looking outside of yourself for contentment. You begin to realize that peace can only come from within your soul; it cannot be found in the external world. It is only through cultivating this space of being that you stop needing, wanting, or craving things in the external world.

Life's challenges can serve as a great opportunity to cultivate a space of being in your life. When I am being tested and challenged, I usually instinctively turn inward to self-reflect. If you are able to spend the majority of your time in deep reflection and contemplation, you will be able to carefully examine the many barriers that have stopped you from connecting to your soul. The more you learn to connect to the inner radiance stored deep within your soul, through a state of simply being, the more you realize you have enough—and thus become perfectly content and peaceful. When you connect with this inner treasure, you realize that you are perfect just as you are and that life is perfect just as it is. You realize that you always have everything you need.

Stillness

Stillness is the natural outcome of turning within and being internal. This quiet and still space of being allows you to not only connect with your soul and receive the divine presence of Spirit, but also allows you to access your intuition. Your intuition is the "gut feeling" that you get about things. Without fail, it tells you what you should do next, how you should do it, and in what context. Your intuition, in the words of a Native American elder I once spoke to, is "the map that the Creator gave you so you would not get lost." Intuition is your spiritual radar, which helps you to successfully navigate your way through the turbulent waters of life. This spiritual radar becomes stronger the more you quiet your mind and still your body. It cannot be felt when you feel pulled outside of yourself in endless distractions. It only becomes clear when you have achieved a state of inner peace and stillness.

This state of inner peace and stillness is best cultivated through silence. Silence is the necessary ingredient for unfolding a peaceful and still presence that is attuned to the great mysteries of being alive. In Mother Teresa's eloquent words, "We need to find God, and He cannot be found in noise and restlessness. God is the friend of silence. See how nature—trees, flowers, grass—all grow in silence; see the stars, the moon and the sun, how they move in silence.... We need silence to be able to touch souls."

Only through silence can you create the outer conditions for your inner world to open up and reveal your soul-space. To achieve this space, it is necessary to remove all the outer "noise" from your life. This means decluttering your life and removing all the distractions that stop you from going inward and being still and silent. For me, these distractions can always be reflected by my mental space. When I am not in my soul-space, I always find myself spinning around in circles of thoughts about the most futile things. These thoughts force me to talk too much, plan too much, do too much, and worry too much. They force me out of the present moment and cause me to be disconnected from my true nature. The fourteenth-century Persian poet Hafiz illustrates this in his poem entitled *Curfews:*

> Noise
> Is a cruel ruler
>
> Who is always imposing
> Curfews,
>
> While
> Stillness and quiet
> Break open the vintage
> Bottles,
>
> Awake the real
> Band.

When I was going through my cancer treatments, I often felt like an experiment that was continually being poked and prodded. I would get woken up at four in the morning for vitals, five in the morning for blood work, six in the morning for breakfast, and on and on. I felt so completely overwhelmed from the chaos that oftentimes it would get very difficult to connect with a space of silence and stillness. When the doctor would come in to tell me what decision I needed to make next, I barely even questioned it. I was so far removed from my inner truth and my intuition that I had allowed the doctors to make all my decisions for me.

Gradually, I started to feel empty inside, without a purpose. The chaos of my situation had left me unable to feel calm and peaceful inside. I had felt so distracted by the nurses going in and out of my room, the doctors telling me to do this and that, and the endless stream of phone calls, that I was unable to relax and connect with myself. And then a question occurred to me: how was I ever going to heal myself with all this chaos and noise continually surrounding me?

The next week, since my time in the hospital was over, I intuitively felt that what I most needed was time to be quiet and still. I decided to go on a retreat and spend a week by myself—with no distractions. This time alone was not only necessary after what I had just been through, but was also one of the most enlightening weeks of my life. On the first day of the retreat, I wrote this short poem in which I asked myself if I would be able to go inward, quiet my mind, and learn how to relax again:

> *Silence and Stillness*
> *Reveal your essence*
> *Do nothing but rest*
> *This is your test*
> *Can you set aside*
> *All your worries*
> *And all your problems*
> *And look deep inside?*
> *Can you forget*
> *All the anxiety*
> *Buried inside your mind*
> *And live within*
> *Holy time?*

Can you give yourself away
To seeing the beauty
Of this perfect day
And experience the everlasting peace
Of the Divine?

During this week, I eventually started to come back to myself. Every day was spent in silence and stillness—and as time progressed, I gradually began to feel more calm, more centered, and more at ease in myself. The silence that surrounded me, even though at first it was a little overwhelming, had begun to nurture my entire being. I no longer felt empty—instead I felt whole. I no longer felt scattered—instead I felt calm. I no longer felt upset and confused—instead I felt perfectly clear. I spent the entire week listening to what I had to say, how I felt, and what I thought. My inner voice—my intuition—had become clear again. The many questions and concerns about my health I had now answered, by simply being quiet and still. By spending this precious time listening to, respecting, and honoring myself, I quickly delivered myself out of the chaos of my situation and back into the home and sanctuary of my inner truth.

Once again in the words of Rumi, "Only let the moving waters calm down, and the sun and moon will be reflected on the surface of your being." I love this quote because it truly defines the power of stillness. By being still, you remove every barrier that stops you from witnessing the absolute perfection of who and what you are. When you remove all these unnecessary barriers (in the form of all the "noisy" distractions) you will be able to fully experience the radiance of your soul. With this connection to your soul, you will be able to respond to life without any confusion about yourself and your life. You always know the truth. You always feel the truth. You always are connected to your intuition, which is the inner bridge that connects you to your soul and allows you to be in continual contact with your inner world.

This soul-based connection liberates you from the heavy burden of fear and confusion, and all the unnecessary distractions that come with that burden, and allows you the freedom to truly live your life. Again, the words of Deepak Chopra ring true: "What is freedom? Freedom comes from the experiential knowledge of our true nature, which is already free. It comes from finding out that our real essence is the joyful field of infinite consciousness that animates all of creation. To have the experience of that silent witness is just to be. Then we are free."

With this newfound freedom, you will be able to approach your life with a deeply soulful presence. This presence will provide you with the still and serene inner space that allows you to witness the absolute brilliance of your true nature. The more you see the radiance of your true nature, the more you will live your life in continual awe and wonder at the overwhelming beauty and divinity that lives inside and all around you.

Simplicity

Simplicity is the way of life that unfolds from nurturing a space of being in your life. A simple way of life naturally brings harmony, balance, and patience. These three qualities stem from the many important inner realizations that you have already developed on your healing journey. They are the direct outcome of having worked through the previous six gateways. While in the previous gateways you have awakened to these life-changing realizations, at the seventh gateway you refine and develop them even further. This is done through a practice of mindfulness. This mindfulness is the tool that continues to help you work through the complexities of resistance and fear. Since your healing journey is always evolving and because you are always in a continual process of becoming, you never truly arrive at a place where you do not have to face the complexities of resistance and fear. What does happen, though, is you learn how to "catch yourself" quicker and quicker and bring yourself back to the present moment. This catching yourself helps you to release these complexities through a precise and meticulous moment-to-moment awareness, and brings you quickly and gracefully back into an uplifted, inspired, and simple way of life.

To be simple means to be completely pure and genuine, without any doubt, fear, or anxiety. Complexity only arises when you become tainted by a lack of wholesome and harmonious intentions—and thereby susceptible to fear-based responses that aren't aligned with your highest self and your highest good. These habitual patterns, such as addictions, obsessions, and neurotic tendencies, force you to be impure and inauthentic with the present moment, forcing you to escape rather than to engage, to fight rather than to relax, to struggle rather than to let go. Simplicity, on the other hand, allows you to engage with the present moment and with life in a genuine and honest manner.

Harmony, balance, and patience—which all comprise a simple and divine life—support your ability to sustain this uplifted and peaceful presence that is devoted to being pure and genuine in every thought, word, and action. I will now explain these three aspects in further detail.

The first aspect, harmony, unfolds through the understanding that, in the words of the ancient sages: "You are that!" This understanding, which I have previously described in this chapter, helps you to realize that there is no separation between yourself and anything else. You realize that you are in all things, and all things are in you. This helps you to achieve an inner harmony, because you realize that you have everything you need and that there is nothing ever to strive for or accomplish—the whole universe exists in your very being.

The second aspect, balance, unfolds through the understanding that you are perfect, just as you are. This realization, which I further described in the Trust chapter, allows you to not get out of control by pursuing futile desires and attachments that force you into living

OPEN UP THE GATES
Of grace
That fills you
As endless light
Fills the stars
And gather this light
And pray
That you may
Be reborn
To breathe every breath
With compassion
To turn every moment
Into a blessing
To open your heart
To the serenity
Of your own self worth
And in this awakening
You give birth
To an inner space
Of peace and stillness
Where you feel yourself
As complete silence
As pure consciousness
As overflowing bliss

in an extreme and unbalanced way. Because you have connected to the perfection of your soul, you no longer feel the need to pursue unhealthy attachments to drugs, food, work, or whatever it may be, to make you feel better about yourself. Inwardly you already feel whole and perfect, because you are in touch with the enduring and timeless wisdom of your soul.

The third aspect, patience, unfolds through the understanding that life is perfect, just as it is. This realization allows you to stop needlessly worrying about your situation in life, because inwardly you know that it is how it should be—that there are no accidents. You understand that each and every situation that you face has a grand design within it and all you ever need to do is simply allow it to unfold. This allows you to spend your time focused on the process of life rather than worrying about the product. If you are obsessed about the outcome or goal of everything you do, you wind up never enjoying your life. You also wind up holding on too tightly, unable to give yourself away to your experiences. In order to fully let go, you must trust the power of life with every ounce of your being. Through this unwavering focus, you develop an extremely flexible and patient attitude, because you always know that, in the words of the poet Rainer Maria Rilke, "Life is in the right, always."

Simplicity instantly rids yourself of every fear-based response, every anxiety-based tension, every unnecessary and burdensome struggle that gets in the way of your connection to life. It does this by keeping you continually in tune with the cosmos. The truth is that the universe and nature all operate through simplicity. Nature never struggles to achieve the next season—it naturally unfolds. Nature never forces fruit to ripen—it simply happens. Nature never tries to quickly turn day into night, anxious or worried about the outcome—it gradually changes. There is never any force or struggle in nature— so why should you struggle?

When I took the weeklong retreat by myself, as mentioned in the last section, I was completely surrounded by the beauty of nature, and it was the sole reason I was able to return to myself. By observing the ease and simplicity in nature, I was able to begin to nurture an ease and simplicity in myself. By going for walks in the mountains, sitting by rushing rivers, and listening to the glorious sounds all around me, I instantly cleansed myself of all my anxiety and stress. It would have been almost impossible for me to hold on to such unsettled, uneasy feelings amongst the peace and harmony that surrounded me.

During one of my many walks that I took that week, I came to a very old bridge that stood over a gorgeous river. The bridge was covered with many vines and there was an abundance of different wildflowers surrounding the banks of the river. Before I even took one step onto the bridge, I stared at this beautiful scene of nature in complete awe and amazement. Right as I stopped, a raven flew over my head and landed on the bridge, staring into my eyes, for what seemed like an eternity. This experience was the pinnacle of my healing experiences that week. Before I went on that walk, I had felt so tormented from the past year of cancer treatments and was completely at odds with how I was going to persevere. The beauty of nature quickly helped me realize that I had everything I needed to heal. All I needed to do was listen, observe, and then receive the enormous beauty that surrounded me. I wrote a poem the following day, after this experience, that described what I went through. It is entitled "The Raven":

> *The bridge stands before me*
> *Dark steps linger*
> *In the midst of memories*
> *Like misty clouds surrounding me*
> *I can't seem to move*
> *But then the raven arrives…*
>
> *I feel the dark passage before me*
> *Shadows upon shadows*
> *Whispering fearful secrets*
> *And I begin to imagine*
> *A joyful and untouchable landscape*
> *That I once visited…*
>
> *The silence erupts through*
> *This bird's ancient eyes*
> *And I envision my pristine dreams*
> *Open and present*

Calling me inwards
To remember how it used to be
Before the pain—

I can't stop staring into
The raven's mystical eyes
Knowing I am not alone
Knowing that this passage
Is necessary
For me to be delivered
Into the infinite land
Of possibility—

So I take each difficult step
I breathe each difficult breath
And I forget each darkened thought
And allow this bridge before me
To open and lead me home

The power and beauty of nature is an invaluable guide to help cultivate simplicity in your life. This is because by spending time in nature, you begin to see that you are not separate from nature. You realize that nature is what you are—if nature is full of harmony, balance, and patience, then so are you. This realization brings you to a full understanding of your true nature and allows you the freedom to stop struggling with unnecessary complexities. The more you give yourself to this pure and genuine way of simplicity, the more perfectly at peace and content you will become.

How to Enter this Gateway: Experience Peace

When your heart is filled to the brim with life, it will overflow with peace. Peace and contentment are the natural outcome when you engage in every aspect of life—embracing and beholding every precious moment. This grateful and open state of being awakens your soul and opens your heart to receive the blessing of your divine self.

Your divine self is always grateful for life, grateful for each and every experience, no matter what it entails. Even though your divine self still experiences suffering as a natural part of the life process, it no longer struggles. There is never any struggle because your divine self knows the true reality—that you are not separate from Spirit or God—and because you realize that you are not separate from God, you feel free to receive the great mystery of life with open arms.

At this last and final gateway, where you enter the peaceful realm of your soul, all you need to do to enter is to simply experience the great bliss of your being. All this gateway entails is that you simply be. Since you have peeled every thick and heavy layer that has covered your core, all you need to do now is stare and marvel at its beauty—listen and hear its great song—feel and be enveloped by its enormous radiance.

I can remember a very important day in my healing journey with cancer when I felt as if I broke through the many barriers inside myself and allowed the healing presence of my soul to shine through. It was a beautiful summer day and I was lying on my bed feeling quite sick. I could hear children in the street outside playing and laughing. I could feel the afternoon sun starting to peek through my bedroom window. I heard people going about their days, walking down the street, or riding in their cars. Feeling extremely forlorn because I felt separate from all of this, I started crying because I no longer felt a part of life. I began to feel as if I was isolated from everything that was good in the world. So I wearily and achingly got up from my bed, put down the book I was reading, and went onto my front porch. As soon as I stepped outside, I felt as if the brightness of the sun cast away the heavy darkness inside me, and then I felt as if this overwhelming warmth penetrated every cell of my being. I sat down on my porch, closed my eyes, and never felt so peaceful before in my life. Instead of feeling broken and separate, I felt unbelievably whole and perfect. In just one moment, I had changed my entire mood. I started to cry again, because I began to realize how perfect and beautiful all of life was and how it was only my own fearful barrier of self-pity that was stopping this feeling from coming through. I intuitively stood up and placed my hands together in the prayer position and bowed to the entire universe. When I went back to my bed to lie down, I opened my book to read the words of Morihei Ueshiba, the great Aikido Master and author of *The Art of Peace*, "When you bow deeply to the universe, it bows back."

It only takes one moment to peel the thick layers of self that hide the core of your being and feel the warmth of the eternal sun. This warmth flows from the healing space of your soul, the healing space of God. When you are enveloped in this great warmth, you begin to feel that you no longer need anything—that you have every-thing—because you realize you are everything. It is this very feeling, this innate wisdom, that arises from your soul, that gives birth to inner peace and contentment.

The experience of peace unfolds by allowing the bliss-ful presence of your soul to make every pore tingle, every cell dance—every inch of your body feels an awakened presence of divinity—and then allowing it to flower from within. This blossoming of divine love and peace is your birthright. It is what you have come here to do. At the seventh gateway, you unfold this awakened presence through spending time in nature, cultivating stillness and simplicity, and using your time to silently meditate on your highest self. Again in Morihei Ueshiba's words, "You are here for no other purpose than to realize your inner divinity and manifest your inner enlightenment. Foster peace in your own life and then apply the Art to all that you encounter."

This "inner enlightenment" bestows you with the blessing of being impeccably present, fearlessly open, and compassionately in love—with all of life. How is it possible to struggle when you feel this way? How is it possible to not turn the experience of a challenge into a great awakening? How is it possible to not awaken your divine potential? How is it possible to not realize your highest self and generate an infinite wellspring of miracles and blessings?

Through your deeply spiritual presence, you now experience yourself as perfectly whole and complete. It is through this feeling that you become physically, mentally, emotionally, and spiritually healed. Through this feeling, you unfold your highest divinity and foster peace in every aspect of your life.

Exercise: Working with Mantras

The experience of peace and contentment unfolds from an inner realization of your divine and spiritual nature. Once you are fully connected to your soul—to your divine and spiritual nature—you experience life in a completely new way. This awakening of Spirit transforms your whole experience of life. With your soul awakened, you no longer struggle with yourself or with life. With your soul awakened, you continually give yourself away to love.

As I have already discussed, the way to allow this transformation space to grow is through the cultivation of silence and stillness. Silence and stillness relax the mind and body, which then allows you to access the inner realm of your soul. One of the best ways to quiet your mind and body and allow the light of your soul to shine through is through the use of mantra. As I described in the Spirit chapter, mantras are simply a prayer stated out loud. They are frequently repeated verbally or silently over and over again, which allows you to immerse and lose yourself in the feeling and vibration of the mantra.

This next exercise will use a mantra to help you to not only fully relax your body and mind, but also allow you to witness the inner presence of divinity. This exercise is best done outside in nature. If this is not possible, a quiet room in front of your personal altar will work just fine.

The mantra we will be using originates from India and is called the "So'ham" mantra. This mantra means: "I am that." The "So" of the mantra means "I am" and the "ham" of the mantra means "that." In this mantra, the word "that" refers to Spirit. The meaning of this statement is that there is no separation between you and Spirit—you come from and exist within the same divine perfection as all of God's creation. Also, this mantra is considered to be the most "perfect" mantra, because it naturally reflects the sound and vibration of the breath, which makes the sounds "so" and "hum."

As you are sitting down, either in front of your altar or outside in nature, I would like for you to practice being silent for five minutes with your eyes closed. Remember to sit with an upright yet relaxed posture. During this time, allow all of your internal "noise" to leave you. Use your breath to let go of any extraneous thoughts by "breathing them out" of you. This is done by releasing all unnecessary noise of the mind through the exhale of your breath. On each exhale, I would like for you to make your breath more audible, as well as drawing it out for a longer duration of time, so that you allow all extraneous thoughts to be released.

After you have sat in silence in your "inner sanctuary" for at least five minutes, releasing all internal noise, you can then start practicing the mantra. Continue to keep your eyes closed. Begin by mentally repeating "so" on your in-breath and "hum" on your out-breath. You can use the sound of the breath to help create the internal sound of the mantra. While you practice this mantra, observe the inner and outer flow of your breath. Feel this inner flow as the divine presence of Spirit inside you. Lose yourself in this flow. Allow yourself to witness the miraculous presence of bliss, love, and Spirit that lives inside you. Allow the flow of your breath to become absolutely effortless. Continue practicing this exercise for at least ten to fifteen minutes.

The Message of this Gateway: Simply Be

By connecting to the ecstasy and bliss of your soul, you feel yourself as what you truly are—Spirit. You realize that your physical reality can be directly influenced and harmonized by this spiritual presence. You realize that all you have to do is turn inward and experience this inner radiance. It is this inner radiance—of the soul and of God—that will nourish you in every way imaginable.

By visiting this temple of peace inside, you allow yourself the freedom to simply be. This is because you feel that you no longer need anything. You experience everything inside of yourself. You feel the entire universe residing in your being. There is nothing to ever search for outside of yourself, because you no longer feel a separation between the external and internal world. You experience the world in perfect harmony. You experience yourself as part of this harmony. You feel divinity in yourself and in all of creation and are content to simply be and witness this miraculous unfolding.

Quiet friend who has come so far,
feel how your breathing makes more space
    around you.
Let this darkness be a bell tower
and you the bell. As you ring,

what batters you becomes your strength.
Move back and forth into the change.
What is it like, such intensity of pain?
If the drink is bitter, turn yourself to wine.

In this uncontainable night,
be the mystery at the crossroads of your senses,
the meaning discovered there.

And if the world has ceased to hear you,
say to the silent earth: I flow.
To the rushing water, speak: I am.

—Rainer Maria Rilke

Bibliography

Anthony, Carol, and Hanna Moog. *Healing Yourself the Cosmic Way.* Stow, MA: Anthony Publishing Company, 2006.

Barrows, Anita, and Joanna Macy. *In Praise of Mortality.* New York: Riverhead Books, 2005.

Braden, Gregg. *The Divine Matrix: Bridging Time, Space, Miracles, and Belief.* Carlsbad, CA: Hay House Publishers, 2007.

Campbell, Joseph. *Reflections on the Art of Living: A Joseph Campbell Companion.* Edited by Diane K. Osbon. New York: HarperCollins Publishers, 1991.

———. *The Hero with a Thousand Faces.* New York: Princeton University Press, 1973.

Castaneda, Carlos. *The Teachings of Don Juan: A Yaqui Way of Knowledge.* Berkeley and Los Angeles, CA: University of California Press, 1969.

Chodron, Pema. *Taking the Leap: Freeing Ourselves from Old Habits and Fears*. Boston: Shambhala Publications, 2009.

———. *When Things Fall Apart*. Boston: Shambhala Publications, 1997.

Chopra, Deepak. *Power, Freedom, and Grace*. San Rafael, CA: Amber-Allen Publishing, 2006.

Cousins, Norman. *Anatomy of an Illness*. Boston: W.W. Norton and Company, 1979.

Dossey, Larry. *Healing Words*. New York: HarperCollins Publishers, 1993.

Durckheim, Karlfried Graf. *The Way of Transformation*. Sandpoint, ID: Morning Light Press, 2007.

———. *Hara*. Rochester, VT: Inner Traditions, 2004.

Dyer, Wayne W. *The Power of Intention*. Carlsbad, CA: Hay House Publishers, 2004.

———. *Your Sacred Self*. New York: HarperCollins Publishers, 1995.

Emoto, Masaru. *Hidden Messages in Water*. Hillsboro, OR: Beyond Words Publishing, 2004.

Foundation For Inner Peace. *A Course in Miracles*. Mill Valley, CA: A Course in Miracles International, 1992.

Frankl, Viktor. *Man's Search for Meaning*. Boston: Beacon Press, 1992.

Gibran, Kahlil. *Wisdom of Gibran*. Edited by Joseph Sheban. New York: Philosophical Library, 1966.

Goldberg, Natalie. *Writing Down the Bones*. Boston: Shambhala Publications, 1986.

Hanh, Thich Nhat. *The Heart of the Buddha's Teaching*. New York: Broadway Books, 1998.

Hay, Louise. *You Can Heal Your Life*. Carlsbad, CA: Hay House Publishers, 1984.

Hesse, Hermann. *Siddhartha*. New York: New Directions Publishing Corporation, 1951.

Ilibagiza, Immaculée. *Left to Tell: Discovering God Amidst the Rwandan Holocaust*. Carlsbad, CA: Hay House Publishers, 2006.

Ingram, Catherine. *Passionate Presence: Experiencing the Seven Qualities of Awakened Awarenesss.* New York: Penguin, 2004.

Ladinsky, Daniel. *The Gift: Poems by Hafiz*. New York: Penguin Books, 1999.

LeShan, Lawrence. *You Can Fight for Your Life.* New York: M. Evans and Company, 1977.

Levine, Peter A. *Healing Trauma: A Pioneering Program for Restoring the Wisdom of Your Body.* Boulder, CO: Sounds True, 2005.

Pert, Candace. *Molecules of Emotion.* New York: Simon and Schuster, 1997.

Regardie, Israel. *The Art of True Healing*. Novato, CA: New World Library, 1997. Ed. Marc Allen.

Remen, Rachel Naomi. *Kitchen Table Wisdom*. New York: Riverhead Books, 1996.

Rilke, Rainer Maria. *Letters to a Young Poet.* New York: Norton and Co., 2004.

Ruiz, Don Miguel. *The Four Agreements*. San Rafael, CA: Amber-Allen Publishing, 1997.

———. *The Voice of Knowledge*. San Rafael, CA: Amber-Allen Publishing, 2004.

Rumi, Jalal al-Din. *The Essential Rumi.* Translated by Coleman Barks. New York: HarperCollins Publishers, 1996.

———. *The Illuminated Rumi.* Translated by Coleman Barks. New York: Broadway Books, 1997

Samuels, Michael. *Healing with the Mind's Eye*. New York: Simon and Schuster, 1990.

Sherwood, Keith. *The Art of Spiritual Healing*. St. Paul, MN: Llewellyn Publications, 1987.

Siegel, Bernie and Barbara Siegel. *Spiritual Aspects of the Healing Arts:* Chapter 4 from *Spiritual Aspects of the Healing Arts*. Compiled by Dora Kunz. Wheaton, IL: The Theosophical Publishing House, 1985.

Tolkien, J. R. R. *The Lord of the Rings.* New York: Ballantine Books, 1973.

Trungpa, Chogyam. *The Path is the Goal.* Boston: Shambhala Publications, 1995.

————. *Shambhala: The Sacred Path of the Warrior.* Boston: Shambhala Publications, 1984.

Ueshiba, Morihei. *The Art of Peace.* Translated by John Stevens. Boston: Shambhala Publications, 1992.

Williamson, Marianne. *A Return to Love.* New York: HarperCollins Publishers, 1992.

————. *The Gift of Change.* New York: HarperCollins Publishers, 2004.

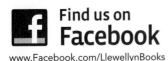
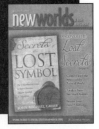

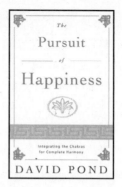

THE PURSUIT OF HAPPINESS
Integrating the Chakras for Complete Harmony
DAVID POND

Many people today need guidance in finding fulfillment in our often-disconnected world. Human beings are complex, but the secret to experiencing happiness is simple—you need only to look within.

David Pond, author of the bestselling *Chakras for Beginners*, offers an easy-to-follow system for manifesting true happiness in your life. Pond describes all seven dimensions from which we experience life—physical identity, emotions, willpower, heart center, thought patterns and intuition, imagination, and spirituality—and gives practical methods for developing and integrating all levels. Focus your attention, seek clarity with meditation and breathing, ground your energy, fine-tune your emotional intelligence, cultivate stronger relationships—and much more.

Transcending religion and accessible to everyone, this seven-step program shows you how to overcome everyday challenges, achieve a healthy balance, be a better partner and friend, and create a richer and fuller life.

978-0-7387-1403-5
264 pp., 5³⁄₁₆ x 8 $15.95

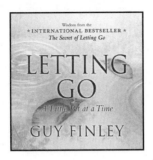

Letting Go

A Little Bit at a Time

Guy Finley

With more than 200,000 copies sold, Guy Finley's international bestseller *The Secret of Letting Go* has touched people around the world. Now the best of Finley's message of hope and self-liberation is available in an attractive gift-book format.

This portable treasury of wisdom from Llewellyn's bestselling self-help book presents an empowering quote for each day of the year. It features a new introduction by the author, inspirational photos, and comes in a handy take-anywhere size. *Letting Go: A Little Bit at a Time* makes it easy to let go of fear and reach a new kind of self-understanding that leads to true happiness.

978-0-7387-1432-5
384 pp., 4¼ x 4¼ $9.95

TO ORDER, CALL 1-877-NEW-WRLD
Prices subject to change without notice
Order at Llewellyn.com 24 hours a day, 7 days a week!

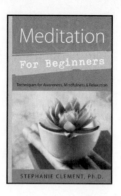

MEDITATION FOR BEGINNERS
Techniques for Awareness, Mindfulness & Relaxation
STEPHANIE CLEMENT, PH.D.

Award Winner!

Break the barrier between your conscious and unconscious minds.

Perhaps the greatest boundary we set for ourselves is the one between the conscious and less conscious parts of our own minds. We all need a way to gain deeper understanding of what goes on inside our minds when we are awake, asleep, or just not paying attention. Meditation is one way to pay attention long enough to find out.

Meditation for Beginners explores many different ways to meditate—including kundalini yoga, walking meditation, dream meditation, tarot meditations, and healing meditation—and offers a step-by-step approach to meditation, with exercises that introduce you to the rich possibilities of this age-old spiritual practice. Improve concentration, relax your body quickly and easily, work with your natural healing ability, and enhance performance in sports and other activities. Just a few minutes each day is all that's needed.

978-0-7387-0203-2
264 pp., 5³⁄₁₆ x 8 $13.95

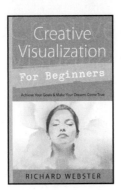

CREATIVE VISUALIZATION FOR BEGINNERS
Achieve Your Goals & Make Your Dreams Come True
RICHARD WEBSTER

Everyone has the natural ability to visualize success, but ordinary methods used to reach fulfillment can be inefficient and unclear. Creative visualization allows anyone to change the direction of his or her life by mentally picturing and altering images of their goals. In his popular conversational style, bestselling author Richard Webster explains the methodology behind creative visualization, and provides readers with the tools and knowledge necessary to achieve their goals in all areas of life, including business, health, self-improvement, relationships, and nurturing and restoring the soul.

Creative Visualization for Beginners includes simple exercises enhanced by real-life situations from the author's personal experiences with creative visualization, and demonstrates how to react when you encounter difficulties along the way. In addition, he gives advice on what to do if you have no predetermined goals in mind, and how to implement positive results while maintaining your natural balance.

978-0-7387-0807-2
264 pp., 5³⁄₁₆ x 8 $12.95

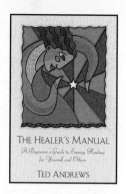

THE HEALER'S MANUAL
A Beginner's Guide to Energy Healing for Yourself and Others
TED ANDREWS

Noted healer Ted Andrews believes it is our unbalanced or blocked emotions, attitudes, and thoughts that deplete our natural physical energies and make us more susceptible to illness. *The Healer's Manual* shows specific ways—involving color, sound, fragrance, herbs, and gemstones—to restore the natural flow of energy. Use the simple techniques in this book to activate healing, alleviate aches and pains, and become the healthy person you're meant to be.

978-0-87542-007-3
264 pp., 6 x 9 $14.95